Dance and Other Expressive Art Therapies

When Words are Not Enough

Edited by
Fran J. Levy, Ed.D., B.C.D., C.S.W., ADTR

with
Judith Pines Fried, M.A., ADTR and
Fern Leventhal, M.A., ADTR

Routledge
New York & London

Published in 1995 by

Routledge
29 West 35th Street
New York, NY 10001

Published in Great Britain in 1995 by

Routledge
11 New Fetter Lane
London EC4P 4EE

Copyright ©1995 by Routledge

Printed in the United States of America

Library of Congress Cataloging-in-Publication Data

Dance and other expressive art therapies: when words are not enough /
    edited by Fran J. Levy.
        p.   cm.
    Includes bibliographical references and index.
    ISBN 0-415-91228-8. — ISBN 0-415-91229-6 (pbk.)
        1. Dance therapy. 2. Movement therapy. 3. Dance therapy for
    children. 4. Movement therapy for children. I. Levy, Fran J.
    RC489.D3D34 1995
    616.89′ 1655—dc20   95-16839
                                                             CIP

To our patients, students, and colleagues.

Contents

Contents

Part 2 / Children

Foreword

Anyone who works with individuals through the healing arts knows the complexity of human nature and the diversity of human needs. As a clinician and educator for almost thirty years, I have come to appreciate, more so than ever, the power of movement to illuminate, clarify, and heal.

In the chapters that follow, the reader is offered a unique opportunity to enter the clinical setting, and to participate in the healing process with both the patient and the therapist. The field of dance/movement therapy has long awaited a book, such as this one, which gives us detailed clinical material on specific patient populations. Fran Levy's first book, *Dance/Movement Therapy: A Healing Art*, provided a strong practical, historical, and theoretical foundation on which this book firmly stands. All of the selections that follow have been written by recognized leaders and contributors to the field.

Expressed in language that appeals to the heart as well as the mind, the book addresses immediate and pressing clinical concerns. Technical jargon is kept to a minimum, and, when used, is always defined. Throughout the book, the needs of patients are carefully considered and creatively met through the courage and perseverance of each therapist. Thoughtful and sensitive descriptions of the individuals discussed allows for an unusual intimacy between the reader and the patient. The authors believe that the experience of movement, on both symbolic and expressive levels, can transform individuals and guide their journeys to recovery.

Some people can dance what they dare not express in words: their sadness, rage, guilt, and loss; their love and empathy; their wishes, dreams, and often their hidden strengths and courage. In essence, these dances are the language of the body, a language with which to communicate to oneself and to others, the language of illumination and transformation. The moving individual, propelled by thoughts and feelings, hides no more.

Dance and movements, perhaps more than any other medium, go beyond intellectualization and reach deeply into the soul. The chapters that follow vividly describe this powerful process, through short- and long-term treatment, through individual and group work, and in private practice and institutional settings. It is rare for a clinical book to cover such a broad range of therapeutic styles and patient needs. The scope of knowledge and specific areas of expertise displayed by the authors gives us an unusually comprehensive picture of dance/movement therapy.

The first chapter offers an inspirational case study of a young woman suffering from a unique form of multiple personality disorder. This compelling study combines symbolic realization with dance and art, and begins the book powerfully. As the chapters unfold, we are struck by the endless creativity and resourcefulness of both the therapists and the individuals they treat. They find, as did Isadora Duncan, "the divine expression of the human spirit through the medium of the body's movements." (1927, p. 72) Each chapter carries us into dimensions of nonverbal experience that will not be easily forgotten.

Miriam Roskin Berger, ADTR
Director, Program in Dance Education, New York University
President, American Dance Therapy Association

Preface

Socrates wrote, "The examined life is the only life worth living." There is always more to learn about human development and how best to help people. There are many theories. Each sheds light on one corner of a huge dark interior we have come to call the personality. No single theory can tell the entire story and many theories come and go in and out of favor.

No matter the theory, clinical experience does teach us that each individual who comes to therapy presents a unique set of problems, experiences, and needs, in the same way that each arrives with a unique set of fingerprints. No single theory or method of treatment can possibly help all individuals.

Although this notion may seem obvious, too often we unwittingly try to fit our patients into a preformed mold that conforms to what we, as students and therapists-in-training, were taught. In many instances what we have learned may serve us well but not all individuals can or should be put into the same mold. At times we must reach beyond our areas of comfort and familiarity to meet the special needs of another.

Individuals come to us not only with their own unique set of problems but also with a unique set of talents and predilections for different modes of communication and expression. For this reason, it is helpful for us, as therapists, to become comfortable with alternate mediums of expression. Some individuals may be tactile or physically oriented, whereas others may be intellectual or auditory. How individuals experience and organize their thoughts, feelings, and memories needs to be considered in deciding how best to reach them. If we cannot help individuals examine their own lives through the medium that best expresses their internal experience, the examination will remain superficial.

The arts can bypass defensive intellectualization, can move toward uncovering underlying psychodynamics, and can meet specific nonverbal needs. In order for this to happen, however, the most important ingredient is the therapist's openness to, and empathy with, the patient. Through empathy individuals receive the message that they are not alone but are traveling with the therapist in a joint journey of self-examination. It is within this empathic and spontaneous dance between therapist and patient that healing occurs.

Fran J. Levy, Ed.D., B.C.D., C.S.W., ADTR
Brooklyn, New York
April 1995

Sidney Levy, Ph.D.
Professor Emeritus, New York University
April 1995

Acknowledgments

The editors would like to thank the many people who helped in the preparation of this book. For their scholarly suggestions and generous sharing of information, we want to thank the original members of our Editorial Board: Dr. Miriam Roskin Berger, President of the American Dance Therapy Association and Director of Dance Education at New York University; Sharon Goodill, Director of the Dance Therapy Program at Hahnemann University; Dr. Robert Landy, Director of the Graduate Drama Therapy Department at New York University; Dr. Sidney Levy, Professor Emeritus, New York University; Dr. Carmen Michael, Clinical Professor of Psychology at the University of Texas; Dr. James Murphy, Founder and Director of the Frontiers Institute; Dr. Amy Schaffer, Psychologist, lecturer, and author; and Dr. Robert Siroka, Director of The Psychodrama Training Institute in New York City. All of these remarkable individuals played an important role in helping this project get off the ground. Their substantial assistance and belief in the importance of this book are deeply appreciated.

We are also sincerely grateful for the thought-provoking contributions of our Editorial Consultants: Lou Cannon, Dr. Deborah Fried, Jonathan Fried, Marjorie Forrest, Dr. Harry H. Levy, Barbara Melson, Anne Mitcheltree, Dr. Nancy Schulman, and Judith Weiss. Their thoughtful ideas and probing questions were an invaluable contribution.

There were also many Directors of Graduate Programs in Dance Therapy and other Expressive Therapies, as well as prominent dance therapy educators, who took time out of their busy schedules to support the completion of this book and share with us their expertise: Dr. Cynthia Berrol, Dance/Movement Therapy at California State University, Hayward; Dr. Joan Chodorow, author of Dance Therapy and Depth Psychology; Dr. Nana Sue Koch, Director of the Hunter College Dance Therapy Program; Susan Loman, Director of Dance Movement Therapy at Antioch/New England Graduate School; Dr. Irma Dosamantes, Director of Dance Movement Therapy at The University of California, Los Angeles; Dr. Christine Caldwell, Director of the Somatic Psychology Department at Naropa Institute; Dr. Vivien Marcow-Speiser, Co-Program Director for Creative Arts in Learning and Meg Chang, Coordinator of The Dance Movement Therapy Specialization at Lesley College; Arlynne Stark, former Director of the Goucher College Dance Therapy Program and former president of the American Dance Therapy Association; Abbey Cassell; Coordinator of Hunter College Dance Therapy/Social Work Dual Program; Jane Wilson Downes, Graduate Liberal Studies Program at Wesleyan College; Maria-Luise Oberem, a dance therapist in Germany; Dr. Helen Payne, Director of Dance Therapy at Hertfordshire College in England; Dr. Frances Kaplan, Director of The Art Therapy Program at Hofstra University; and, Jane Ganet Sigel, Coordinator, and Barbara Cargill, teacher, of Dance Therapy at Columbia College in Chicago. To these special individuals whose contributions are endless and who take on the difficult challenge of bringing the art therapies to new generations of professionals every year, we are indebted and in awe.

And, to our esteemed colleagues—major leaders in the field of dance therapy—who shared with us their extensive knowledge, clinical insights, and creativity throughout the development of the book, we want to thank: Sarah Becker for her contributions to the growth of dance therapy with multiple-personality-disordered patients; Dr. Eleanor Dipalma, Valorie Zagelbaum and Maria Rubino for their contributions in the area of the developmentally delayed; Amy Soscia Artes, Dr. Anne Krantz, Dr. Danielle Fraenkel, and Barbara Reese, in the area of eating disorders; Dr. Beth Kalish-Weiss for her numerous contributions to the field of dance therapy with special children; Dr. Warren Lett, for his many contributions to the study of multimodal psychotherapy in Australia; Dr. Penny Lewis for her countless theoretical and practical contributions to the field; Bonnie Meekums, for her work with children and abuse; Shira Musicant for her creativity in the clinical use of Authentic Movement; and Dr. Ilene Serlin for her scholarly work developing a movement language for diagnosis and treatment.

Finally, our very special and very patient computer consultant, Robert Yachnowitz, deserves a round of applause for helping us to unravel the mysteries of computer life. His work was complemented by a very warm and wonderful neighborhood professional, Yvonne Claudio, at Computer Tyme in Park Slope. We also want to thank our families for their warm support, encouragement, and patience. And last, but far from least, we want to thank the authors of the chapters that follow; their thoughtful contributions, clinical perseverance, and deep respect for the needs of their patients makes their work rich and unforgettable.

Introduction

Since time immemorial we have understood that words alone are not enough to express the totality of experience. The arts, a source of both celebration and release, have helped us to say what we could not say in words. We sing the blues; we dance out frustration and rage; we jump for joy, reach for love; and we paint the anguish of loss and war. Many dance therapists have heard their patients say that only when they move do they feel. This sentiment is understood among dancers and athletes as well and is echoed in contemporary culture, in a growing interest in nonverbal expression and a recognition of the extraordinary interaction of body and mind, feeling, and form.

Dance/movement therapy, a modality that had its beginnings in the 1940s, is based on the premise that mind and body are inseparable, that what is experienced in the mind is also experienced in the body. This book is a compilation of 16 chapters by pioneering clinicians and educators representing dance therapy and other expressive modalities. Each author presents case information depicting a unique set of problems that continually challenge the therapists.* Underlying the thinking of the authors is the premise that self-expression facilitates personal growth and change and that verbalization alone, unaccompa-

---

*The names and identifying information of all patients have been
changed to protect the privacy of the individuals discussed.

1

nied by affect, creativity, or motor action, cannot touch the full range of human feeling.

The first chapter, a longitudinal study of a young woman who experiences herself as having multiple personalities, points to several major themes. These themes recur throughout the book. The first, though not unique to dance therapy, is the importance of trust, acceptance, and safety within the therapeutic relationship, that is, the establishment of a genuine empathic communication between therapist and patient, as illustrated in Fried's chapter on two children born blind. The struggles of developing such a relationship and its importance are also discussed in the chapters on autism by Erfer and Loman. In Blau and Reicher's work with children at risk of attachment disorders, they discuss methods that promote nonverbal communication between parent and child and the obstacles that commonly interfere in such interactions.

Without a foundation of trust and empathy, meaningful exploration cannot occur. Levy and Baum, in their chapter on multiple personality disorder, point to the difficulty of establishing trust. All of the authors depict the countless ways in which they are challenged to respond both verbally and nonverbally to their patient's needs. Several of the clinical examples are discussed in great detail. The reader is given a chance to experience the development of the therapeutic relationship and the challenges that continually threaten this delicate interaction. What makes these chapters most compelling is the degree to which the therapeutic relationships described involve nonverbal and symbolic communication.

A second theme is the integration of the other art forms—singing, music, drawing, mask-making, poetry, costuming, and performance—all within the treatment process. In itself, each art medium provides an important avenue for self-expression, as is well understood by art therapists, drama therapists, and psychodramatists, and poetry and music therapists. When the arts are used in combination, each medium can enhance, and may contribute new meaning to, the total experience. The dance therapists who contributed to this book frequently augment their movement work by incorporating one or more additional art forms at significant moments in treatment. This theme is emphasized in Levy's work. Her patient, initially too inhibited to make use of movement, finds meaningful expression in other art forms. These experiences eventually culminate in dance. Lawlor, utilizing her patient's natural artistic ability, encourages the making of masks, which are then interpreted through dance. And Harvey, in his work with a sexually abused little girl, integrates play, drama, and art with movement so that his patient can creatively dramatize her feelings. When an individual's body is frozen from trauma, drawing can sometimes pave the way for full body expression.

When additional art forms are introduced into the dance therapy process, they are designed to extend and clarify that which is expressed nonverbally.

Fried uses movement in combination with song to help one blind child grieve the loss of her mother. Duggan, in her work with learning-disabled adolescents, discovered the importance of providing a structure that included specific dance steps, music, costumes, and performance.

Another important theme is the therapists' work with symbol and metaphor, as poignantly illustrated by Murray-Lane and Rose, in their chapters on addiction; Kierr, in her work with anxiety and depression; and Bernstein, in her chapter on sexually abused women. These chapters are rich with case illustrations.

All therapists recognize the profound importance of symbolic communication. The verbal therapist may emphasize the metaphors implicit in dream work and free association. Creative arts therapists, in general, shed light on symbolism through the active shaping of thoughts and feelings that underlie communication. The dance therapist places special emphasis on encouraging dramatic movement metaphors that express the hidden and symbolic aspects of the self. This emphasis on creative and symbolic expression of different parts of the self, illuminates the close connection often made between dance and drama.

Interventions that encourage creative nonverbal exploration are especially helpful to individuals who have been abused or traumatized and whose feelings are inaccessible through words. The dance therapist does not require the verbalization of feelings and memories. Through projective techniques creative arts therapists allow for an aesthetic distance from core emotions while still encouraging genuine self-expression (Landy, 1994). Some therapists believe that survivors can live healthy lives, free of inhibitions, rage, and guilt, only by directly re-experiencing their traumatic pasts. In this regard, Baum dicusses the phenomenon of abreaction in dance therapy. In contrast, a fundamental point emphasized by Chang and Leventhal, in their chapter on battered women, is that dance and movement alone can mobilize individuals to overcome incapacitating fear and isolation. This belief is undercored by Sandel and Scott–Hollander in their work with the elderly.

The roles that the dance therapist plays vary as each therapist adapts to individual needs. Many move with their patients in supportive and mirroring roles, whereas others act essentially as empathic observers. Occasionally, some therapists do their own dances in order to reflect back to the patient, or group, what they perceive, or as a way to help the group feel more comfortable with movement. This method is discussed in Lavender and Sobelman's work with borderline individuals.

There are always a complex set of reasons why a therapist chooses a given mode of interaction. In the case material that follows the authors clarify not only what they do, but why and how. They reflect aloud on their work, bringing the reader along as a co-therapist. At times the authors write openly about their mistakes, for example, overinterpreting a movement or becoming involved in a difficult countertransference.

The book is divided into two sections: adults and children. In the section on adults, emphasis is on exploring the insights that come from creative expression. In the section on children, the emphasis is more on the child's experience in the moment. For both groups finding a meaningful realm of communication presents the greatest challenge and the deepest reward. In both sections, creativity and movement are powerful sources of inspiration and self-affirmation.

Although this book is organized around specific patient groups, it is not intended to pigeonhole a particular group of people with any single set of methods. Each person is different and treatment decisions should always be individualized. The chapters that follow tell stories of treatment in which clinicians help individuals to follow a creative impulse until it finds full, meaningful expression. In their efforts to bring people out of isolation, into reality and into a deeper communication with themselves and others, each therapist emphasizes a unique perspective on dance and other expressive art therapies.

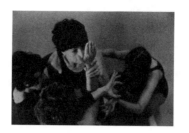

Part 1

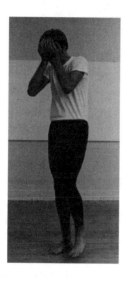

Adults

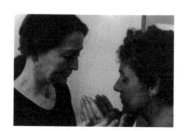

1

Nameless: A Case of Multiplicity

Fran J. Levy

The following chapter discusses the long-term treatment of a young, highly intelligent, professional woman who, in addition to severe anxiety and depression, suffers from a unique form of multiplicity. The therapy process presented unusual challenges and demands that had to be considered in every stage of the treatment. Although the patient was seen three and sometimes four times a week, the treatment was not psychoanalysis. It was psychodynamically oriented, however, and the interventions used were within the realm of a creative arts or multimodal approach to psychotherapy. The intensity and style of treatment were always determined by the presenting problems and the unusual developmental needs of the patient.[1]

Multiplicity

It is common for us to speak of ourselves as though we were divided into parts. "Part of me is happy but another part is lonely and sad." "Part of me is mad at my parents but another part understands their limitations." "At times I feel torn apart." Such phrases are commonplace, but what does this language that refers to parts of the self really mean? Are we actually divided into distinct parts? Or is the word "part" a metaphor for conflicting and repressed feelings? If we are actually divided within ourselves, what is the impact of this division? And finally, how can we as therapists engage our patients' many parts into meaningful dialogue? In this chapter, the case of Rachel is intended to shed light on both the complex issues that contribute to fragmentation of the self and on the creative, symbolic, and empathic interventions required for the gradual unification of the self.

The term used to identify a state of fragmentation is "multiplicity" and the definition of the term includes a range from mild, imperceptible splits to distinct, discrete identities that alternate in their control of the self, that is, multiple personality disorder or MPD (Beahrs, 1982). In order for the case of Rachel and the concept of multiplicity to be understood, it is useful to look briefly at child development, particularly at issues of separation/individuation.

Separation/Individuation and the Development of Self

The birth of a child may be viewed as a two-stage process. Initially there is the actual birth, when the child makes its physiological separation from the mother. This birth is delineated in time and space. The second birth, which takes an unspecified amount of time and varies with each individual, is the child's psychological birth and is referred to by Mahler as the process of separation–individuation (Mahler, Pine, & Bergman, 1975).

Mahler explains that having been in the womb, attached to the mother for 9 months, after birth the infant continues to feel attached, still at one with the mother, undifferentiated. When the baby is in utero there is a constant stream of biochemical information and stimuli that largely originate in the mother but is also experienced by the infant. After birth there is a change in the communication from mother to infant. The way the mother holds, looks at, and talks to the baby, her tone of voice, her gentle or rough touch, all contribute to the communication. Infants continue to feel that they are an integral part of the mother, and some feeling of emotional, physical, and intellectual connectedness continues throughout the individual's life.

All individuals mature at different rates and, although a person may become a successful adult, success does not mean that the person is fully individuated. Few of us, in fact, are either wholly attached or completely distinct. Instead, each of us falls somewhere on a complex continuum between the two extremes. The more one is attached, however, the greater the experience of fragmentation and, conversely, the more one experiences oneself as distinct from others, the greater the sense of integration (S. Levy, personal communication, May 4, 1993).

Causes of Multiplicity

There is no single cause of multiplicity. Instead, there are numerous possible causes that, when joined together, could lead to the perception of one's self as multiple.

One cause of multiplicity may be incomplete separation from parental figures. Feelings of attachment and connectedness are universal and are not necessarily dangerous to the integrity of the self. The degree to which an attachment is unhealthy can be determined by the degree to which any individual is able or unable to maintain independent thoughts, feelings, and actions. Extreme unresolved attachment to a parent may leave a person unduly vulnerable to the influence of others. Individuals with such attachments may perceive another as physically part of them. They may feel divided, torn between themselves and the other by whom they feel controlled and from whom they cannot differentiate. Because such individuals are unable to know where they end and another begins, all relationships present a potential threat to the integrity of the self.

Another cause of multiplicity may stem from the fact that we often carry into adulthood the fragments of earlier, immature selves (Freud, 1960). Popular literature refers to these fragments as "our inner selves," or as our secret "baby" parts (Missildine, 1963). For some, such fragments are well integrated and therefore insignificant in their influence on the personality. For others, the fragments can be threatening, especially if they are ignored. In advanced stages of fragmentation, an individual may be split into distinct personalities, each with fully developed and independent needs, beliefs, memories, even illnesses (Braun, 1986; Kluft, 1983; Putnam, 1989). The personalities may alternate in their jurisdiction over the entire system of selves. When such is the case, we refer to these selves as alternate personalities, not fragments. Alternate personalities or "alters" represent a high level of organization and their etiology expands beyond, but does not exclude, incomplete separation/individuation. Individuals split in this way are diagnosed as having multiple personality disorder (MPD).

Some theorists speculating on the etiology of multiple personality trace the development of separate distinct personalities to an early childhood experience of severe and often protracted abuse. The abuse may be physical or it may be psychological. Either form can lead to a marked arrest in development in which parts of the individual split off and become alters as a way of protecting the self (Braun, 1986; Kluft, 1983; Putnam, 1989). Some of these same theorists also point to the possibility that certain individuals may be born with a biochemical predisposition toward alternating ego states or varying states of consciousness.

An important criterion that differentiates severe cases of MPD from milder forms of multiplicity is the degree to which an individual's different selves are conscious of each other. When there is little or no "co-consciousness" the diagnosis is clearly multiple personality disorder. If, however, the individual is aware of other selves and has the ability to negotiate life decisions with some degree of communication with the organizing or "host" self, the diagnosis may fall more within the realm of multiplicity or mild MPD (Beahrs, 1982).

The Arts and Multiplicity

Throughout history artists, philosophers, and scientists have understood the inherent limitations of verbal language to express all nuances of life. Therapists who work with the creative arts provide their patients with an opportunity to find an expressive language that is most natural and meaningful to them and most central to their nature. The arts allow individuals to speak through different media and the medium that is used should reflect the patient's needs in the moment. If we accept as fact that we carry pieces of our childhood with us, it is easy to understand why a variety of expressive modalities can help to elicit and clarify nonverbal experiences. We know that children tell us many things through play, art, dance, and music that they may not be able to say in words. It follows that adults, carrying aspects of their childhood with them, can also benefit from creative symbolic action.

As will be seen in the case of Rachel, a combination of movement, drawing, writing, music, and symbolic realization gave expression to both the child and the infant Rachel had within. To keep Rachel solely in a verbal mode of expression would have limited her ability to experience and nurture the very young parts of herself, the parts she came to call "The Kids." In addition, because Rachel had not been allowed to express herself verbally as a child, she had stored many of her early feelings in art and symbol. In order for her to find these parts of herself, a number of expressive and symbolic activities were incorporated in her treatment.

As creative-art therapists we have a unique set of tools, which, when used intelligently and empathicly, help us to reach deeply into the complex weave of the human personality. By the same token, used carelessly, or without a genuine understanding and empathy for the multileveled needs of the individual, the same tools can create further fragmentation and chaos.

The Case of Rachel

Background

Rachel is a bright, psychologically astute career woman. After she became comfortable in treatment, she showed herself to be highly articulate. Her superior intelligence was apparent throughout the therapy, through our interactions, her responses to treatment, and through her ability to work in a creative and symbolic fashion. The following history was collected over a period of many years. It is comprised of Rachel's memories of her childhood together with material learned from communication with family members.

Rachel was the first born in an intact family. She had two younger brothers, 2 and 6 years her junior. Rachel said that "the boys" were her parents' favorites and that after their birth she felt ignored and like a misfit in the family. From age 7, Rachel was often left home with her mother to clean house while the boys went on "boy trips" with her father. When she went out with the family on weekends, it was often to watch the boys play ball. She believed that her mother had contempt for her and for girls in general. She recalls that her mother constantly criticized her—a memory confirmed by her brothers. "She was yelled at all the time for no reason. She was a quiet kid. We could see how sad she was. We were all afraid of our mother but Rachel got the worst of it."

As a child Rachel was withdrawn, basically afraid of asserting herself with anyone. Trying to be "good," she was always neat and clean, methodical, attentive to detail, and a good student. "You simply couldn't be any other way in my mother's house. Whatever my mother said, that was the way it was. Rachel reported that her mother often told her what a wonderful family she had and how lucky Rachel was to have this family. Rachel always believed her mother and this belief is what puzzled her. How could she be so unhappy in such a wonderful family? "Something must be very wrong with me" she thought.

Rachel's mother had severe mood swings that included unpredictable bursts of rage. As a result, Rachel "walked on eggshells" and was "always on the lookout to see what her mood was" so she would know how to behave. When she helped her mother in the kitchen and didn't move fast enough, her mother shoved her out of the way and berated her for being "too slow." Her mother frequently threatened to "smash" her.

Rachel remembers being shy, awkward, and overweight from the time of elementary school, always uncomfortable with herself and others. She tried hard to be pleasing but felt that nothing she did could win her mother's approval. By the time she was in high school she stopped believing that she had a wonderful family. She began to hate her mother and wanted "nothing to do with her."

Making friends was understandably difficult for Rachel. "How could I feel good enough about myself to make friends when my mother made me feel like nothing? I had no self. I was a nobody. The friends I did make she criticized. She accused me of running after them and letting them use me." Rachel recognized that she did let people "walk all over her." She knew that she did it partially to win their affection and because she was afraid to speak up.

As far back as second grade, Rachel remembered looking to her female teachers as surrogate mothers. This tendency continued throughout high school. In college, however, Rachel made a "best friend" and they were inseparable. Her mother harshly ridiculed her friend and accused Rachel of being a lesbian. The accusation was deeply upsetting to Rachel whose sexuality at this time was unformed.

In spite of her struggles throughout childhood, Rachel managed to complete her college education with honors. In addition, by the time I met her she had a good position on Wall Street. Despite this evidence of success, she still felt "like a nobody," hating her life and herself. She believed she had become professionally what her parents wanted but not what she wanted. She had once dreamed of becoming a psychotherapist and had wanted to study psychology in college but had been discouraged by her parents who pushed all of the children into business. "You simply didn't go against them." Rachel hated the way women were treated in business. Her experience as a woman on Wall Street was reminiscent of her childhood experience. She felt left out of the "old boys club," "different," "invisible."

When Rachel came to treatment she said "I can't stand living like a nobody anymore." She wanted to be free from her mother's domination and from her feelings of self-hatred. She also recounted numerous somatic complaints she believed were part of "being uptight." As long as she could remember she suffered from frequent stomachaches, headaches, and insomnia. She had a fear of flying so intense that it precipitated cold sweats and heart palpitations. Off and on Rachel had flirted with the idea of suicide.

Initial Sessions

Rachel first came to see me 12 years ago. She was a tall, somewhat overweight young woman, neat, clean, and on time. She stood anxiously with her head bent over, hands nervously fidgeting and shoulders raised with tension. Her speech was quiet and at times inaudible. I asked her if she'd like to sit down. She did, but after sitting briefly, got up and began to pace back and forth. The studio was a large carpeted space with chairs, large pillows, and play things. Rachel had plenty of room in which to walk back and forth. As she paced, her high-pitched speech was tense, childlike, and self-conscious. She asked several times if I wanted her to leave and wondered if she was "too much" for me. She seemed irritable. Rachel was clearly uncomfortable face to face; she was unable to sustain eye contact. Sitting across from me appeared to be an excruciatingly painful experience. She was like an animal behind bars. Eventually she described herself in just this way. "I feel like a caged animal, like I'm in a prison." Pacing was a way to both contain and express her tension. Due to the degree of anxiety she was experiencing, we decided in the first session that she would come in twice a week. Later in treatment our contacts increased.

Approximately two weeks into treatment, aware that words were frustrating for Rachel and aware that she was not ready for expressive movement, I asked Rachel if she would like to draw. We sat together on the carpet but Rachel did not pick up the crayons. Instead, she did something she had not done before. She glanced up at me with a mischievous twinkle in her eye. On what seemed an impulse, she picked up the crayons and playfully threw them at me, looked down and laughed. I also laughed, paused silently for a moment and threw them back at her. We laughed together for the first time and Rachel's tension was momentarily released. The seeds of spontaneity were planted. I gradually learned that rapport through play and symbolic communication were what Rachel needed. Trust was most difficult for Rachel. Through her playfulness she had opened the door a little. From this point on, she let me know in countless ways that keeping the doors of trust open would be a constant challenge.

Because Rachel was both tense and disconnected from her body, I needed to find areas of self-expression that did not depend solely on either verbalization or body movement. As mentioned above, Rachel is extremely bright and eventually became articulate about herself, her upbringing, and her needs. In time, with extensive input from Rachel, I learned what intermediary activities would help her become more comfortable with herself: drawing, writing stories about drawings, visualization, "symbolic realization"[2] (Sechehaye, 1951), play, music, and, most importantly, humor. All of these activities were possible long before movement was part of our work.

Rachel's Earliest Drawings

Rachel's first drawings, done in the third week of treatment, provided a look into her dynamics at that time and presented graphic indicators of the concepts discussed above: attachment, fragmentation, separation/individuation, and multiplicity. They also illustrated her ability to handle her complex thoughts and feelings—her multiplicity—through strong obsessive/compulsive defenses.

Drawings are projective tools from which we can draw certain hypotheses about how individuals see themselves and what dynamic conflicts may be influencing their behavior, ideation, and feelings. Drawings are a means through which an individual can unconsciously tell the therapist important things that may not be accessible in words. Like spontaneous movement, drawings help people project into the outside world something of what they experience inside. Because Rachel was unable to move expressively, drawing was important as an intermediary modality.

The science of projective drawing began in the 1940s and since that time has become a well-established method of diagnosis and assessment (Abt & Bellak, 1950; Hammer, 1958; Machover, 1949). The interpretations of Rachel's artwork are derived primarily from the pioneering work on figure and animal drawing analysis done by Dr. Sidney Levy[3] (1950, 1958, personal communications, 1980–1994). Although drawings can serve as a useful springboard to expressive movement, mobilizing images prematurely may bring individuals into contact with parts of themselves, or feeling states, they cannot handle. The analysis of drawings and their use for facilitating movement is best done by someone well trained in both projective methods.

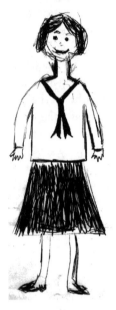

Figure 1: First Figure Drawing—Our Hero

Rachel's first drawing was of a female figure (see Figure 1). About this figure, she wrote: "This is our hero, that for this moment will remain nameless. Her age depends on the given circumstances at any one time. Our hero (will I be my own hero) works on Wall Street and her appearance is just that of others in her environs....She likes what she has on because it reminds her of the Van Trapp kids from The Sound of Music....the scene where the Father blows his whistle and all the kids come down the stairs and fall in line" in their uniforms.

As suggested by the word "nameless," Rachel's story indicates that her identity is diffuse. Lack of identity, however, should not be mistaken for weakness of character; this is a nameless "hero." When she wonders if in the future she will become her "own hero," she speaks of a wish to be independent and in command of herself. But for now she is just like all "others in her environs." In other words, she experiences little distinction between herself and others and, perhaps, feels that she is not completely separate from her surroundings. In addition, she experiences her identity as continually shifting "depending on the given circumstances at any one time." She also is controlled by parental figures. She reacts to the sound of the Father's whistle, as do all of the other, as of now, indistinguishable children in their identical uniforms. For the moment Rachel's inner selves are unidentified. They are dressed alike, but each is a different age, representing a different stage of her own development.

It was after she made this drawing that Rachel, for the first time, identified the baby self she came to call Nameless. Over the next six months the baby gradually emerged as a distinct alternate personality with the perceptions, feelings, speech patterns, and all the needs of a developing child.

In examining the drawing itself, the first question to be asked is what stands out most strongly? What is the first impression of the figure? The drawing, done by an adult, looks like a child, who does not appear at ease in her body. Pronounced graphic constriction around the neck, drawn long, narrow, and with excessive stroking, suggests trying to keep mind and body separate.

Perhaps she fears being flooded with emotions. The heavy stroking of the skirt is another indication of anxiety over bodily feelings. The drawing's attentiveness to detail suggests the potential for a methodical approach to solving problems and strong obsessive-compulsive defenses. The control evident in Rachel's drawings could also be seen in her limited and self-conscious use of her body. Both the constricted motility and tense drawing warned me to be cautious in the area of expressive movement. The overall tone of the drawing is one of intense inner struggle. Strong defenses have been necessary to help her contain the tendency toward fragmentation.

After the figure drawing, I suggested that Rachel draw an animal (see Figure 2). Her narration about the duck she drew is as follows: "This duck, believe it or not, has a friend, a cat, that lives on one of the streets here in a place called something like 'Far from the Ordinary.' The cat is red and looks like a lion...." In her story Rachel symbolically tells of the 'others' she experiences as part of her self, a cat and a lion. It again appears that she

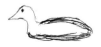

Figure 2: Flat Animal Drawing—"A Nameless Female Duck"

does not experience herself as having a single identity. Instead her identity is an amalgam of possibilities. Interestingly, the cat and the lion have more defined and distinct personalities than the duck. A duck is a fairly innocuous, nonthreatening animal. The cat and the lion, on the other hand, are predators. The changing character of the animal illustrates a plasticity in her own identity. The story was prophetic in that it suggested what I could expect from Rachel in the future, when she began to feel more comfortable in treatment.

The repeated stroking of the body of the duck can be seen as a question: Where do my body boundaries end and yours begin? In animal/and/figure drawing analysis, multiple lines executed in this way may be indications that the artist experiences herself as attached to others instead of as a separate, distinct, and intact self. The multiple lines often play a double role, which is unconscious to the drawer. They are at once an expression of the presence of others within the self and a defense against intrusion from the outside. As in the drawing of Our Hero, the multiple lines are her attempt to keep her selves under control.

This extensive explanation of Rachel's drawings is meant to clarify the correlation between issues of separation/individuation and the concept of multiplicity. Rachel's drawings enabled a deeper understanding of this fascinating phenomena and also introduced me, in another way, to this most interesting young woman.

Rachel entered my office feeling that she was different from other people. She felt as though she were an odd duck who lived in a place "far from the ordinary." How far from the ordinary was this place really? What took place in all the years of treatment and where is she today? These, and many other questions and answers, will be discussed in the following pages.

"Nameless"

Although Rachel's early figure and animal drawings pointed in the direction of multiplicity and even possible multiple personality disorder, Rachel did not present alternate personalities during the first 2 months of treatment. In retrospect, her anxious pacing may have been expressive of the childlike feelings that were struggling to be released but were as yet unidentified.

Rachel told me that Nameless first took conscious shape in her thoughts when, after seeing her drawings, I asked if she could give her figure drawing a name. She paused, thought about my question, and said, "Yes, Nameless."

At first Rachel only described Nameless' feelings and needs in a general way: "Nameless is cranky" or "Nameless is tired, she needs you." Later she began to talk about Nameless in more concrete terms—what Nameless did at home, the hour Nameless went to bed, the clothing she wore, and the activities she enjoyed. When I asked Rachel if she actually saw Nameless in the room with us, she said, "I see her in my mind."

Nameless' existence in treatment was expressed primarily through Rachel. She was spoken of in the third person: "Nameless needs to nurse." "Nameless is lonely." "Nameless is wearing her cute pink overalls." Within 3 months after Nameless emerged, her needs had become central in our sessions. If Rachel wanted to talk about her problems at work, Nameless gave her only so much time before she became visibly uncomfortable and irritable. Nameless made it evident whenever she was tired of "grown up talk."

In the beginning, as reported above, Rachel paced back and forth during sessions. Three weeks after she revealed Nameless, she was able to find a place that was comfortable for both of them. She curled up on a long cushion in a fetal position close beside me, sometimes facing me and sometimes with her back to me. This was safer for her than sitting across from me, the position that risked eye contact. To be truly herself in our relationship, Rachel needed a physical posture in keeping with her stage of development, and, at this time, Rachel was most often Nameless, the baby, rather than Rachel, the successful adult.

Finding a position and location from which Rachel and Nameless could engage in treatment was complicated by Rachel's occasional fear that she had a bad odor and that I would think she was dirty. These fears were projections of her feelings of shame—feelings that were also expressed in physical rigidity, fear of eye contact, and her initial difficulty in verbalizing. She was embarrassed, in fact, about all of her physical functions: nose blowing, sniffing, sneezing, going to the bathroom. She did not allow herself to do any of these in our sessions for many years. It was 10 years before she allowed herself to use my office bathroom.

If Rachel accidentally touched me, the drive to merge was triggered and she immediately became anxious. One day she handed me a drawing and in the process touched my hand. At once, she needed to be reassured that she had done nothing wrong.

Later in treatment Rachel struggled with how she could avoid eye contact and still receive what she needed from me. Because the eyes provide one of the earliest senses through which the infant takes in the mother, it was important for Rachel to allow Nameless to see her therapy/mom. Such looking caused her great anxiety, however. Rachel resolved her conflict by asking me to close my eyes while Nameless looked at me. When asked why she wanted my eyes closed, Rachel explained that Nameless was embarrassed by the depth of her "need for a mommy." Rachel said, "I'm afraid that if you look at me, you'll only see the big me, not Nameless, and you'll think I'm too big and fat to be nursed and held. You'll think this is stupid. You'll laugh at me."

During this time it became clear that Rachel had a real relationship with Nameless. She nurtured Nameless as a mother nurtures a very young child.

Nurturing Nameless: Symbolic Realization

Rachel progressed in treatment from talking about what Nameless was doing, wearing, and thinking, to making specific requests, always in third person. "Can you hold Nameless?" "Can she sit on your lap?" "Can she nurse?"

Knowing that Nameless was an infant, I attended closely to Rachel's requests and spent considerable time trying to determine how best to respond. I reasoned: if Nameless lived in the safety of Rachel's mind, and Rachel was able to reach Nameless through imagery and symbolization, perhaps I could also reach Nameless in this way. Perhaps I could find a way to speak to Nameless with Rachel's help. With this in mind, the next time Rachel said Nameless wanted to be nursed, I responded by saying, "Nameless is nursing now." Then, in a voice that sounded like a very young child, Rachel asked, "Is she in your lap now?" and I said, "Yes, she's in my lap now." None of this was acted out physically. With the help of Rachel's imagination, our dialogue continued:

"Can you hold Nameless?"
"I'm holding Nameless now."
"What are you doing with her?"
"I'm rocking her and stroking her hair."

"Can she look into your eyes?"

"Yes."

"What does she see in your eyes?"

"There is lots of love in them for Nameless."

As our dialogue continued, Rachel's body relaxed and silent tears rolled down her face. Following these nursing sessions, Rachel's speech was more audible and articulate. After many repetitions of such moments, Rachel one day suddenly moved from lying in a fetal position to sitting up. She then unwittingly touched her belly as if to express contentment. As I watched these changes, it was clear that Nameless was making a transition from a hungry, needy infant to a more mature and contented stage of development.

In a particularly significant session Rachel asked, "Would you really hold Nameless?" This was a difficult question for Rachel to ask as she believed herself to be profoundly unlovable. It was also a question I had anticipated and about which I had thought carefully long before she asked. I knew that Rachel's ability to ask for her needs to be met was a positive sign; yet, long-term ramifications for therapy had to be considered. Would it be helpful if I crossed over the line that distinguishes symbolic realization, which takes place through shared imagery, from the actual acting out of fantasy? What would it mean to Rachel? Would it give her what she needed to grow or might it keep her in infancy? Might it seduce her away from trying to manage the difficulties of her adult life? Finally, might she lose all sense of reality and become fixed in a world in which she would experience herself again as the completely dependent, attached baby and the therapist as the all-powerful biological mother instead of the mother surrogate?

Because all of these ideas had already been considered, when the question came I said, "I don't think it would be a good idea for me to hold you in my lap. If I actually hold you, it might keep you a baby and prevent you from growing. I want Nameless to feel loved but I'm also aware of the rest of you and all of your different needs, not just Nameless' needs." I went on to explain, "Touch is very powerful. It could unintentionally constrict you." Rachel listened carefully to my words and seemed to understand that she was safe in her therapist's office and that her therapist would not attempt to either dominate or infantalize her as her mother had.

Even though Rachel's needs were intense, she had an extraordinary intelligence about what was healthy and safe for her. She understood the dangers of being swallowed up by a parental figure and said she was relieved to know that I would nurture her only in a fashion that would be safe.

From our first attempt, it was clear that symbolic communication provided nurturance that was helpful to Nameless. In time, Rachel stopped asking to nurse and began to substitute images of bottle-feeding for breast-feeding. In much the same way as with nursing, I talked Rachel through the images of this more grown up source of nourishment. In time, even the bottle became less important to her and was replaced by symbolic hugs thrown playfully through the air—an activity that made Nameless giggle with joy. As time went on, Nameless also came to enjoy our singing together. She was growing up, weaning herself, and moving from infant to toddler.

Nameless became increasingly comfortable with all of the playful gestures, love sounds, and songs that are typical of a young child's interaction with parents. How, I wondered, was she so receptive to this language of love if she had not received it herself? Had she, somewhere in her past, experienced this quality of attention, perhaps prior to the birth of her brothers and before she attempted to assert her independence, thereby coming into conflict with her parents? Or, did she observe this behavior and take it in while watching her parents with her younger siblings? These questions cannot be answered at this time, but it is clear that she thrived from the experience of reparenting and she knew exactly what she needed.

In order to further Nameless' small developmental steps, activities and structures were needed to provide her with an ongoing sense of security and some anticipation of consistency. Most of Rachel's problems with Nameless centered on difficulty in believing that her therapist/mommy existed and cared about her even when she was not with her. Rachel's hold on reality was sometimes tenuous. It was not uncommon for her to see me in the morning and then leave a message on my answering machine later in the day to say, "Nameless is upset, she can't remember talking with you." Rachel was unable to hold onto a continuous perception of me and the fear of loss was ever present. For this reason, we began to meet three times a week and also had three regular 30-minute phone sessions on the days she did not come to the office. On the seventh day of the week, Rachel had "special permission" to leave a 3-minute message on my answering machine.

This continual need for contact can be explained by Rachel's developmental level at the time she entered treatment. When Nameless was first discovered, it became clear that a large part of Rachel was fixated at an infant and toddler level. In the same way that you would not leave an infant for long periods of time without contact, you also could not leave Nameless. Although Nameless' developmental needs matured significantly as treatment progressed, her need for symbolic, creative, and interactive expression continued throughout treatment.

Building Memories/Decorating the House.   As Nameless matured into a young child, her gains were reflected in Rachel. After 3 years in treatment,

Rachel now spoke more freely of her childhood, and of the emotional and intellectual deprivation she had experienced. Rachel confided that she longed for positive childhood memories. She felt embarrassed about what she perceived to be the bleakness of her past. She told me that the experiences in the "playroom" (Nameless' name for the studio) were beginning to fill in the void of the past. "We're building mommy memories and it makes Nameless feel more like other kids and less envious when she sees families having fun together." During this time in treatment Rachel made an important animal drawing and wrote a story. The animal was a whale named Timothy (See Figure 3).

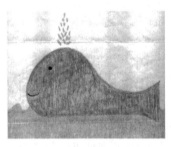

Figure 3: Timothy the Whale

"Timothy is a very happy whale. That's because he has a very nice mommy that loves him a lot. She takes Timothy swimming all over the ocean and shows him all the special spots....Timothy asks a lot of questions about why things are the way they are but Timothy's mommy is very patient and kind so that her baby will learn all about the world. And Timothy's mommy is fun—so much fun that Timothy can hardly sleep at night waiting to play with her.

The amorphous shape of the whale is a symbol of Rachel's internalization of the therapist as "mommy." When compared to the tiny duck and the story of the duck, one sees that she is now feeling full and content. Rachel isn't only receiving food as nourishment, however. Through her attachment to the therapist, she feels that she is also seeing and learning about the world around her in a positive way.

At this time Rachel compared the treatment process to creating a new house. "We're not just tearing down the old house and putting up a new one on a stronger foundation, we're also decorating it." She said that time in the playroom reached her "deep and inside" and formed the foundation of her new house. At home, Rachel wrote down her ideas about building the house. She gave me a copy and put her own copy in her "Love Sounds Box," a little box Rachel said Nameless made to "store her special moments."

Preserving her ideas was one way for Nameless to stay close to her therapy/mom when she was not in the playroom. Drawing and writing enabled Nameless to keep positive experiences with her at all times. It was always difficult for Nameless when Rachel was away from therapy, and when Nameless suffered so did Rachel. "It feels like years since I saw you last—Nameless can't remember you," she would complain, even though at this time our in-person sessions were three and sometimes four times a week.

Many of our activities were now structured specifically to help Nameless feel more connected between sessions. In addition to regular sessions and the 30-minute phone sessions, she also had her own answering machine at my office so she could leave long messages. For a year before she had her own machine, Rachel took a cassette player with her wherever she went and talked into it as if she were having a conversation in the playroom. After she had the new answering machine, her need for the cassette player gradually diminished. She did, however, continue to write in a personal journal and leave regular messages on the new machine.

"Decorating" the house included many activities in which Rachel showed a significant capacity to develop games and images to nurture Nameless. For example, she brought in children's books and asked me to read them. Nameless especially liked books about animals; together we made animal sounds and at times played raucously. She also brought in little toy animals with which to play, and wanted to leave them in the playroom. It was as if she were leaving a part of herself with me, assuring that I would not forget her and would keep a part of her safe.

Another activity was singing together. She enjoyed it when I changed the words so that the lyrics were about her. She loved the lullaby "I Gave My Love a Cherry." The first time I sang it to her was over the phone when I was on vacation and Nameless "couldn't find or remember" me and was in a panic. When she finally did get me on the phone she was extremely withdrawn and it was hard to reach her. I told her that I was holding Nameless and wanted to sing to her. I began to softly sing "I gave my love a cherry that had no stone....I gave my love a story that had no end...." The singing calmed her and whenever she, in the future, was in a "scary state," not able to find me, I usually could contact her with this song. I encouraged Rachel to sing "The Cherry Song" to Nameless whenever Nameless felt she was "losing" me. In her journal Nameless once wrote, "I guess I haven't quite internalized you yet, or what it is that you give to me....I know too that the you I'm trying to internalize is that part I'm missing, and...when I have it, it won't be you anymore but Rachel—a total Rachel."

Session after session we worked with the same themes. Gradually Nameless became able to tolerate longer periods of time away from me. In addition, our activities brought the Nameless part of Rachel out in a more real and physically spontaneous way. She began to giggle and laugh and gradually began to assert more of her own personality into our play.

Even during our most playful moments, Rachel continued to speak of Nameless in the third person. But as she did so, I could hear in her voice the sound of a happy child. I also saw ongoing changes in her body as she engaged more fully in play. Her habitual rigidity began to release and a more childlike spontaneity took over.

Gradually, play was replacing the "bad memories" of the past and Rachel's house was becoming "richer in feeling and more complete."

The Importance of Humor. From the beginning of our work Rachel had trouble with even minute changes in treatment. She became rageful and distrustful at the slightest alteration of the playroom. We had a parting ritual that included blowing two kisses across the room to each other as she left. If I forgot and blew only one kiss, she became anxious and wondered if I did this on purpose and was it a "sign" that I "was changing" and didn't care for her anymore. Rachel reacted by asking me her usual repetitive questions, "Are you mad at me?" "Do you remember me?" or "Are you different today?" Because of the childlike tone of her voice, I knew it was Nameless speaking. The questions were endless. Saying, "No, I'm not mad." or, "Yes, I remember you," were unconvincing to Nameless and at these moments, neither Rachel nor Nameless believed my assurances.

Sometimes I knew my repeated responses became mechanical in tone, and Rachel always knew it too. Asking, "Why do you think I'm mad or have forgotten you?" so irritated Rachel that she only repeated the question. I realized that you cannot ask toddlers to reflect on their feelings. They *are* their feelings.

It was obviously important to find a way to break the repetition of the questions and to interrupt their underlying morbidity. It was also important to be cautious not to be rejecting or aloof. Nameless was never easily placated. But I found a way to respond when the questions came again.

One day when Rachel had asked three times, "Are you mad?" and I said, "No" each time, the fourth time I added cheerfully, "No, but if you ask again, that might change." Sensing she was being played with, Rachel took the bait and asked again. Then, with obviously make-believe anger, I said," I'm not mad. I'm fuuuuuurious!" Rachel repeated,

"You're fuuuuuuurious!?"
"Yes, fuuuuurious!"
"How furious?"
"Very furious!"

"I thought so," Rachel responded with evident self-satisfaction. "At least now you're telling the truth." In the playfulness, we both acknowledged reality.

The exchange brought both Rachel and Nameless out in a manner that allowed for a safe release of aggression without fear of punishment. In addition, it allowed the kind of honest exchange Rachel had not had with her mother and for which she yearned. Through interactions of this kind, Nameless, and therefore Rachel, became more at home with both playfulness and aggression.

It seemed possible at this time to escalate the humor and the playful aggression in our interactions with the aim of freeing Rachel's body and movement patterns and thereby promoting a richer integration of her mind and body. Rachel's movement patterns were still quite constricted even though she was responding more fully to our exchanges. Now, when she asked repeated questions, I gave her "a hard time." In response, she would raise her voice as she giggled and slam her fists on the pillows and try harder and harder to aggravate me. We both accomplished our goals and in the process also enjoyed ourselves.

Now, four years into treatment, it was clear that changes in Nameless were reflected in Rachel's behavior and feelings. When Nameless was happy, Rachel was happy. When Nameless was miserable, so was Rachel. Although there was a definite distinction between them, unlike more extreme cases of multiple personality, they only occasionally acted as completely distinct personalities. Their moods affected each other; Rachel could not be a happy adult until Nameless was a happy child.

"Hannah's Rage." Although a warm and loving disposition was the major part of her personality, Nameless was also prone to rageful withdrawals. Rachel began to reflect on the times when Nameless would slip into states of rage and she was able to identify these rages as resembling those of her mother. Rachel was helped to free herself from these rages by labeling them and talking about how she realized she had taken in some of the "worst parts of my mother." During this time she stopped using the words "my mother." She wanted, she said, to separate herself from her mother's influence. I asked her what name she would like to call her. She said, "Hannah," and explained that she got the idea from the song "Hard Hearted Hannah" and, from this point on, the rage was referred to as "Hannah's rage." Giving her mother and the rage a name helped Rachel separate from the overwhelming anger she experienced as coming from "Hannah."

Rachel started to undo the past through the exploration of new, out-of-the-playroom activities such as biking and nature walks. I encouraged her and viewed her efforts as an essential part of her total growth. Rachel had no memory of recreational activities in which her interests were respected and nurtured. All she remembered were "terrible trips where all Hannah did was complain and the boys got all the attention." During this time Rachel needed to report every detail of what she and Nameless did. She began each session with a statement like, "Nameless couldn't wait to tell you about her biking trip." Supporting her new-found excitement about life was a major theme for this period, which was approximately 5 years into treatment.

Nameless was, at this time, fully a toddler and was curious about everything. Demonstrating her new activities, describing them in detail, and keeping a journal all helped Rachel to feel alive and free her from the constraints of "Hannah's house."

Working with Rachel's Angers at Me

As Rachel became closer to her therapy mom and felt safer, she became more expressive of her feelings. Having lived her formative years in an unstable environment in which she was frightened of her mother's sudden and unpredictable rages, she had not developed a model for constancy or unconditional love. As constant as I tried to be for her, Rachel's history was her reality. She continually expressed the fear that her new mom would "tire of Nameless' endless needs and demands." She feared that I would begin to thwart, tease, and ridicule her as Hannah had. Rachel also feared that I would "change," for no reason at all. One day I would "be different." For years Rachel asked "Are you different today?" "Are you the same as you were yesterday?" "Are you angry at me today?" I knew when she asked these questions that she was trying to find out if she was safe with me.

As stated above, reassuring Rachel was a primary task. She was ever ready to feel rejected and deceived. If I tired of reassuring her, Rachel knew it in an instant, would withdraw and even threaten to leave treatment. Because of these issues of rejection and deception, and because of Rachel's extraordinary sensitivity to me, it was important to be vigilant and honest not only with Rachel but also with myself.

Like so many sensitive, intelligent children who grow up in households in which they cannot predict from moment to moment the ever-changing moods of their parents, Rachel had become overly tuned-in to the moods of those around her. She was aware that she had this sensitivity and believed she had developed it because, she said, "it was the only way that I could survive in Hannah's house."

I knew that if Rachel's negative feelings about Hannah became displaced and transferred onto me, our relationship could be in jeopardy. If the negative transference was not interrupted, but was allowed to solidify, the treatment could not continue. Thus, although genuine reassurance, caring, and empathy were the most significant aspects of treatment, helping her to understand where

her thoughts and feelings came from was also essential. Without real understanding, Rachel's anger at her mother would always be displaced and misdirected, not only at her therapist, but also at others who might remind her of
her mother. To help Rachel understand the origins of her feelings in relation to
me, I asked her over and over, " Who is it that gets tired of you?" "Who 'changes'
on Nameless when she least expects it?" Rachel responded, "Hannah" and then
would go on to discuss her "Hannah memories." These questions usually, but not
always, helped her to differentiate our relationship in the present from her memories and perceptions of "the other mother."

Efforts were continuously made to help Rachel separate out what she came
to call her "bad, scary Hannah feelings" from her "good mommy feelings."
The process of weeding out the negative transference from our relationship was
ongoing. Trying not to sound overly pedantic, I explained to Rachel that it was
inevitable, and even necessary for the success of our work, that she would, at
times, see me as Hannah. I explained that this phenomenon was actually crucial and that only in this way could the past with Hannah unfold in the present
where together we could look at and examine all of her feelings and memories.
Explaining this to Rachel relieved her of the guilt she felt about her periodic
rage at me and made it easier for her to talk about her feelings.

"I Just Closed the Door." When Nameless was angry and in control, "all
hell" threatened to break loose. At home, pots and pans got thrown. At times
she literally could not pull herself off the floor. These more extreme acts, fortunately, were rare. For several years during this period Rachel had, at times, talked
about wanting to hurt herself. An increase in contact seemed to calm her and the
threats never went past the talking phase. One incident was particularly dramatic.

Eight years into Rachel's treatment I was in a leg cast for a few weeks as a
result of a fall. During this period Rachel became especially helpful, opening and
closing doors and fixing the playroom furniture. Rachel also made a toe cover to
go over the cast and decorated it in the image of a yellow-braided little girl she
named "Peggy Sue." All of this reminded her of a time when she was 9 and Hannah
had been sick in bed. Rachel recalled that Hannah had been unusually gentle during this time. She had allowed Rachel, for the only time Rachel ever remembered,
to be close to her and to help her. This had made Rachel believe that she was
finally important to her mother. Ironically, her mother's illness became one of the
only special times that Rachel could recall. The special feeling was short lived. As
soon as Hannah recovered, she "changed" and returned to her "old self."

In one session during this period, I did something that I had done many
times before. I closed the door to the playroom in order to begin. This, how-

ever, was one of the jobs that Rachel had taken over and it held special meaning for Nameless. She became visibly upset and words rushed out, "You don't need me anymore? Why can't I do that? Are you taking things away from me now? Are you going to be different now?"

The incident was so threatening that a distraught Nameless took total control of the session and Rachel was nowhere to be found. I knew at once that I needed Rachel to help me explain to Nameless that closing the door did not mean that I had "changed." I would not become mean and push her away.

While shutting the door seemed a simple act, to Nameless it felt life threatening. Although Rachel said she could recognize the connection between this incident and her past experiences with Hannah, she was unable to separate her feelings. She withdrew into rage and despair and said, "I can't go on like this. This is too painful. I can't separate you from Hannah, it's too hard!" Rachel wanted out.

This incident preceded a weekend when I had to be away at a converence but knew that Nameless needed to be contacted. Because Rachel was being controlled by Nameless and the situation could escalate, I telephoned her. She answered my call in the dry distant voice I always heard when she was emotionally cut off, and in trouble. I responded,

> "How are you doing?"
> "O.K."
> "Do you know who this is?"
> "Who!?"
> "It's me." (Quiet pause) "Nameless, do you remember who I am?"
> "No."
> "Guess who's traveling with me?"
> "Who?"
> "Peggy Sue! She misses you but she's enjoying being in the big city.
> People notice her and talk about her." (Quiet—no response.)

Finally, in exasperation I raised my voice slightly and, in a final appeal, said, "ALL I DID WAS CLOSE THE DOOR!" Nameless was silent. The conference was about to resume and I said good-bye, unsure of the effect of my words.

I did know that in the past Rachel had always had positive responses to honesty in our communications. I hoped that my genuine exasperation would shock her out of the past and bring her back to the present. That night when I checked the answering machine, a message from Rachel said, "I explained to Nameless that all you did was close the door, just like you always did. Nameless was so sure that you didn't want her close to you anymore. It was really awful! When you told me you wore Peggy Sue to the conference and people liked her—you reached Nameless but she couldn't say anything. I repeated what you said over and over again and finally Nameless said to me, 'Really? Did she really wear Peggy Sue to the conference?'"

Rachel was back and, for the moment, the destructive mother memories were in perspective. The "good" and "bad" mothers, who had temporarily merged into one, were now separated. This confluence of perceptions would occur again and again, however.

Rachel was back in her role of helping Nameless and it was time to work with Nameless and Rachel to understand what had happened. She seemed available to explore the feelings aroused by this event. It became clear to her that sometimes she did not know the difference between her mother and me and when that happened, her life, she said, felt like "a black hole. It's like being in another dimension and nothing feels real."

Rachel's anger, however, was not always misdirected. At times she was really angry at me: when a session time had to be changed, when I was away or ill, or when she felt I was not sensitive to her feelings. We began to work on the complicated connections between her real anger and the displaced anger. When I made a "mistake," for example, forgetting something she had told me or not appreciating the depth of her emotions, or if I did anything Nameless didn't like, she lost all contact with her positive feelings for me. At such times I became "all-bad." Rachel's inability to see good and bad, strengths and short-comings in the same person compounded the difficulties of our work.

No matter what the source of her feelings, Rachel needed to know that neither she nor Nameless would be rejected for her thoughts or feelings, and that therapy was the right place for her to express herself. She also learned that although there was no shame in any of her thoughts or feelings, her actions need-ed to be carefully evaluated. Rachel needed to know that she was accepted for all of her, not just the good lovable Nameless but also the deeply troubled Nameless.

The Arrival of F.J. Seven years into treatment Rachel introduced a new little girl into the playroom. She told me she was four or five years old and her name was F.J. F.J., she explained, stood for "Fran Junior." Rachel said that F.J. came because "...of you writing a book.[4] It makes me feel proud to be a woman. If you could do something that important then I could be important too. F.J. is named after you because she wants to grow up and be just like you." F.J. seemed to represent the stage of development in which the child moves beyond seeing the mother as only present to serve the needs of the baby, or as an all-encompassing and nurturing breast. F.J. represents the child who could view the mother also as a role model and who wanted to be "just like" the mother. This change implies the beginnings of separation and maturation in that the child now sees that the mother has another life outside of the mother role, and the child sees that she too will have another role someday that will go beyond just being an attachment to the all-encompassing other.

Rachel, however, described F.J. as follows: "She's very thin and tiny. She's so tiny you can't believe it. She's emaciated. She's hurting really badly. Her hair is all gnarled and she's upset, frazzled. She's very, very sad. I don't know if she'll let you reach her. She won't come to you herself but I will bring her to you."

From this point on, F.J. was often present in our sessions. Nameless continued to be important but Rachel had found a way to separate and encapsulate her new "happy parts" in the persona of Nameless. In contrast, F.J. seemed designed to isolate and hold Rachel's pain and rage—feelings that still threatened to overwhelm her. Rachel was not aware of this initially, but several years after F.J.'s arrival, she said, "I think F.J. was once part of Nameless but she split off so Nameless could remain a loving child and F.J., who was a little older, tried to bear the pain of Hannah for Nameless. If it wasn't for F.J. there wouldn't be a Nameless."

In the beginning F.J. came to sessions through Rachel in the same way Nameless had. Rachel spent many hours describing the anguish F.J. experienced. Nameless was now about 4. The intensity of her needs had diminished and, for now, she took a back seat. Compared to F.J. she seemed fairly well balanced and happy. Although Nameless felt left out because of F.J.'s enormous needs, Rachel said, "Nameless cares about F.J. and wants her to be happy."

Trying to meet F.J.'s needs was difficult. She expressed her lack of trust by retreating into rage. She was, according to Rachel, a frail little girl whose "despair and fury ravaged her tiny body."

For several years F.J. had found countless ways to test my constancy and was especially skilled at setting up tests of my commitment. For example, if the answering machine picked up when she called, she hung up without leaving a message and then was enraged because she couldn't reach me. Sometimes she called in a particularly upset state and, when I answered, she was silent at the other end of the line. I told Rachel many times, "If F.J. doesn't leave me a message or speak to me, I don't know that she's looking for me and I can't help her." It was hard for Rachel to see that, intentional or not, these were traps that inevitably left F.J. feeling even more angry and unloved.

While trying to explore this behavior, Rachel explained, "When the answering machine picks up, F.J. gets so angry that she just hangs up. She thinks you're just playing games with her and don't want to speak to her. F.J. can only wait so long to reach you, and if she has to wait beyond that point she starts to 'lose it.' She thinks you're trying to hurt her. She gets enraged and then she just disappears."

It was especially difficult for Nameless when F.J. was in a "bad state." Nameless was now in love with life and was frightened by how fiercely angry and pained F.J. was. F.J. distracted her from her new goals, which were "to be loving and to play and learn new things."

Clearly, Rachel used her intelligence and methodical nature to separate out and preserve the best parts of Nameless. What was not clear was when the split first took place. Was it a result of Nameless' therapy, or were the rudiments of F.J. planted in Rachel's childhood, when she first attempted to protect the different parts of herself? Rachel had always been an organized and methodical person. The techniques she used to adapt to her demanding adult life and career, while continuing to "take care of the kids" attested to this. "The Tin Can" and "The Yellow Room," described below, further illustrate the organizing strength in Rachel's personality.

The Tin Can.   Rachel reported that at times F.J. was so distraught that she disappeared and both Rachel and Nameless wondered where she had gone. They both missed her. One day Rachel came in and announced sadly, "F.J.'s in a tin can." "Why?" I asked. "That's where she goes when she can't cope and she can't reach you." When F.J. was in this state Rachel was also affected. Rachel could not really separate herself from F.J.'s feelings. When F.J. was in "the can" Rachel felt a sense of loss, an emptiness. The opposite of F.J. being in the can was when she was in total control, causing Rachel to go home and kick and throw things around, to become rageful at small provocation. At times, F.J. was itching for a fight.

The precipitating event that drove F.J. into the tin can was that Rachel's mother became ill. Rachel felt genuine concern for her mother and was surprised at her own reaction. Her anger at her mother seemed to disappear temporarily and she worked hard at "being there" for her. But it took a great toll.

At the outset Rachel hoped that her mother's illness might evolve into a reparative experience for their relationship and during this time she felt more kindly toward her. Rachel was able to see her mother more realistically, and in the present, as opposed to how Rachel had perceived her when she was a child. In her current state Rachel's mother was an ailing and frightened woman, not the "monster" of the past.

In treatment, Rachel had begun to make strides at separating from her mother's domination. But her mother's illness had the effect of pulling her back. It was reminiscent of the earlier time when Rachel was a child and her mother's illness had been so seductive. She became increasingly absorbed by her mother's illness and described feeling a loss of herself. "It's really scary. I feel like I want to keep going to visit her. She seems so helpless. It's tearing me up inside." Rachel was beginning to merge again with Hannah. She recognized the feeling and knew it was a sign of danger for her.

The image of a can where F.J. stayed during much of this period was actually a safe place to keep her. Rachel hated for F.J. to be there and described the experience as similar to a prison. In the end, however, the tin can turned out to be Rachel's attempt at self-medication. It represented a sufficiently safe place in Rachel's mind where she could keep F.J. when F.J.'s feelings threatened to overwhelm Rachel. On the other hand, the tin can was a cold, tight, and uncomfortable place. It smacked both of self-punishment and depersonalization and was possibly a concrete representation of her superego—the part of her that worked hard to keep herself under control at all times.

The Yellow Room. F.J.'s hiding place was the tin can not only during Rachel's mother's illness but afterward, while she was regaining her equilibrium. For about 6 months the tin-can image continued to contain F.J. enough to allow Rachel to function at work. Now, a few months after the crisis of her mother's illness, this uncomfortable symbolic container was no longer needed. Rachel found a better place for F.J. Instead of the can, in her mind's eye, she created an esthetically pleasing "yellow room" where F.J. could comfort herself alone.

Rachel had managed to get past Hannah's illness and was now careful not to over-identify with her mother's problems. She accomplished this partially by making her visits and phone calls briefer and less frequent. F.J. continued to be a major influence and kept Rachel feeling vulnerable and tense. F.J. still did not completely trust me although some small moves in my direction were taking place. Rachel told me, "I think she is trusting you a little more now. She told me she wanted to call you over the weekend to tell you what she was cooking."

Even though F.J. was moving closer to me she still lapsed into dangerous withdrawals. Again, as with Nameless, hours were spent considering how best to consistently reach F.J. and how to foster trust between us. As was often the case, Rachel herself found a solution. "Sometimes you just have to leave her alone when she's really hurting. She can't have you near her until she's more together. Asking her questions just irritates her. You're not reaching her where she needs you, low, deep and inside. She needs to go into the 'yellow room' and be by herself. That's where she cries out loud. When she's ready she'll let you in but you have to whisper. It hurts her ears if you're loud."

After this revelation, F.J. and I whispered together through many sessions and many phone calls. Sometimes the whispers were the soft humming of lullabies. Other times we whispered about her feelings at work or with the new friends she was making. And sometimes we'd whisper about lighthearted things like cooking or shopping. But even whispers were at times like loud voices to F.J. and hurt her ears. When I watched Rachel's body closely I could see when even a whispered voice was painful. When my voice was soft enough to reach her without "hurting her," her shoulders relaxed and the lines in her forehead disappeared. Her fingers, which had been hyperextended while rubbing her brow, would relax and she would start to stroke her body gently.

Rachel remembered that when she was growing up she had not been allowed to cry or lose control. Any display of emotion or lack of "perfection" provoked ridicule by Hannah and humiliation for Rachel. In the yellow room F.J. was able "to find her own safe and quiet place" where she could feel her feelings.

During many months of whispering, F.J. grew calmer and more trusting of me. Eventually the whispers included talk of holding and loving F.J. who seemed comforted by the imagery in the same way that the images of nursing had once nurtured Nameless. But for F.J., asking for attention and affection was an enormous step.

As of this writing, the doors of the yellow room are rarely needed and the can is long forgotten. According to Rachel, F.J. is now about 8 years old and feeling proud of herself. The F.J. part of Rachel is a diligent and meticulous worker on the job and in every other area of Rachel's life. She is also the "smart one" who competes with her male counterparts on Wall Street. She does not let anyone push Rachel or Nameless around. Lengthy discussions about the dynamics at work and Rachel's infrequent visits, and periodic phone calls, with her family provoke material that enable the working through of her past. Rachel says that F.J. is the one who can endure the most discomfort, having learned to cope with Hannah as a child. This answered my earlier question about when F.J. had first came into existence.

"Sanding Down the Infrastructure." In going back over Nameless and F.J.'s evolution, Rachel describes the process of her treatment and growth. "We're sanding down the old infrastructure. It's been slow and painful. I don't think you can do this kind of work quickly. F.J.'s pain has been the hardest part but we couldn't avoid it. It was down there at the bottom of the rubble and until we exposed it and made it better—deep and inside—we couldn't start to build the new house. This house is not like Hannah's house. This house has a strong foundation. It's decorated with happy memories."

Losing Weight. Eleven years into treatment (a year before this writing) Rachel began referring more frequently to Nameless and F.J. as "The Kids." Although they were still distinguishable, there were areas in which the boundaries between Nameless and F.J. seemed to merge. Rachel was becoming a strong, more integrated person. Her role with The Kids continued to be a nurturing one. She enjoyed their company and was proud of "their accomplishments" in therapy. Her drawing of the giraffe (see Figure 4) illustrates great strides in the direction of sep-aration/individuation (note the well-defined boundaries) and foreshadowed her ability to lose weight, which began immediately after the drawing.

Without prompting from me, Rachel decided that she wanted to weigh less. For all the years I had known her, Rachel's weight had remained relatively sta-ble, about 40 pounds overweight. At this time she became concerned that she was beginning to gain and this made her feel "disgusting." As a result she decid-ed to register for a Weight Watchers program. Within 6 months she reached her

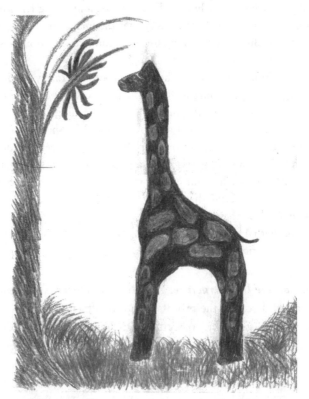

Figure 4: Giraffe Drawing—Predicted a developmental change
and a loss of weight soon to come.

goal of 130 pounds and completely changed her eating habits. During this time she became a dedicated cook and began to enjoy a new, healthy diet.

Interestingly, during the weight-loss period she told me over and over, "I didn't realize how tall I am!" It was as though she was experiencing herself as an adult for the first time. Figure 5, which is of an egret, was drawn after the loss of weight and depicts both her new body image and her growing self-confidence. It also indicates a more integrated sense of self and a greater sense of self-definition. She had literally and figuratively let go of some of her baby selves and relinquished a significant portion of her early attachments.

No longer does she draw round amorphous animals with diffuse boundaries. Her new drawings are larger, stronger, and more centered. The outlines are clear and the overriding feeling is one of self-pride. Her tendency toward multiplicity is still evident, most obviously in the Giraffe (note the many well-defined and distinct vacuoles or "selves"). The time that it took her to draw each individual round circle is a sign of her investment in ordering herself both internally and externally. What is different here is that these selves or parts are drawn in a manner that is well rationalized, organized, and contained. The extreme anxiety of Figure 1 is gone. In addition, she draws herself (the giraffe) almost as big and strong as the tree, a symbol of mother.

For Rachel, the extra weight was likely an expression of her dependent attachment to her parents. She was, in effect, carrying them with her. The weight loss happened quite naturally. When Rachel was ready, she made the decision and set about achieving her goal in her usual methodical manner. Rachel's growth away from her parents and the resultant change in her feelings about herself and her body were plain to see.

Dancing with The Kids. For the first 11 years of treatment the movement interactions between us had been in the realm of play, similar to the play between a parent and a child. The interactions were all age appropriate for "The Kids," and, as such, were nonthreatening. Everything we did helped Rachel become more comfortable and less split off from the many different parts of her. These activities together with the visualization work helped bring Rachel up the developmental ladder. Twelve years into treatment Rachel said Nameless was "about 7 or 8 years old and F.J. about 9 or 10."

Rachel now was strikingly tall, slender, and attractive. At work her friends and colleagues commented on the change they saw in her. Rachel told me, "They say it's not just my weight. They say I seem so much more at ease with myself." She told one of her friends at work that she wished she (Rachel) "could speak up more with the guys when they go after women." Her friend

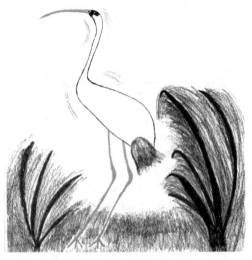

Figure 5: The Egret—Represents a new body
image and self-concept

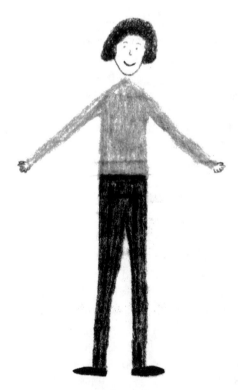

Figure 6: Final Figure Drawing—After loss
of weight—Rachel called this drawing
"a Young Woman"

said, "You do speak up these days. I think they see you as a strong force and are a little intimidated." This new perception shocked and pleased Rachel.

Despite these overt changes, Rachel remained somewhat disconnected from her body. When she stood, it was hard for her to keep her head upright. At times she stooped like a shy child. I often wondered why her emotional growth was not more reflected in her posture and in her general physicality. Isn't the body a reflector of inner thoughts and feelings? How could the new positive feelings she had about herself exist apart from her physical self? Had she not yet fully grown into her new slender body and, if this was the case, how could she be helped to take the next step? Why did her recent drawings indicate a growth that could not yet be seen—the solid, tall giraffe, so proud and satisfied, the slender, attractive, and graceful egret and her last drawing of a person (see Figure 6)? Where were these characteristics in her body?

Rachel told me that the only time she felt connected to her body was when she rode her bicycle. Biking, like other vigorous activities, can stimulate increased bodily sensation and enhance the perception of one's own body boundaries (Schilder, 1950). Rachel described her biking experience "as a feeling of oneness" coupled with a sense of greater autonomy and freedom. This sense of autonomy was new for her, in sharp contrast to earlier feelings of being controlled by others. If a person is excessively attached to and controlled by others, movement can bring about a greater sense of independence.

Rachel explained it this way. "When I first start to ride, I feel awkward, all over the place, not really connected. Then gradually it changes and I feel every part of me falling into place. It's an incredible feeling. Each rotation gets clearer and more precise until I feel completely together."

Rachel knew I was a dance therapist as well as a verbal therapist and had asked to read parts of my book on dance therapy. Like the individuals discussed in the book, Rachel wanted to feel free enough to dance out her emotions. It was unbelievable to her that people could find creative and expressive movements to portray their thoughts and feelings. "Wasn't it embarrassing?" she wondered.

Sometime after her weight loss, Rachel expressed a desire to move in our sessions. I began by introducing simple movements and recognized how extraordinarily awkward and self-conscious she was. I wondered if movement might prove too frustrating and possibly undermine her newly found self-confidence. Were there other ways to help her feel more connected to her body? Perhaps she simply was not "a movement person." On the other hand, her interest in dance therapy, the joy she experienced from our playful movement exchanges, her love of biking and the quality of her art work all told me that expressive movement could be important for her.

In order to test these hypotheses, I tried several approaches. In the past the use of imagery and play had released the spirit of The Kids by giving their needs shape, form, and expression. Perhaps imagery and play could do the same for Rachel's connection to her body. Since Rachel always responded to visualization, it made sense to use imagery as a bridge first to her emotions and then to movement. Knowing she loved birds and knowing the power that animal imagery has to facilitate expressive movement, one day I asked, "How would you move if you were a bird?" She responded, "I can't make that connection. I can't feel movement even though I can see it in my mind." Her response notified me that efforts to bridge mind and body through imagery were not yet possible. She was unable to translate her thoughts, feelings, and images into bodily sensation and action.

Because imagery did not evoke movement for Rachel, another approach was tried. Sometimes a seemingly simple motion like letting the head roll easily in a large circle can provide a temporary release of the mind's control over the body. Rachel put a song on the stereo that she loved. We sat on the floor together and took a moment or so to relax and to try to deepen our breathing. This was not easy for Rachel to do. Then I suggested that she let her head roll from side to side and then around in a circle. I also suggested that she close her eyes, feeling that this might help her to feel more at ease.

I hoped the movement would be pleasurable for Rachel and that she might want to extend the feeling of letting go to other parts of her body. We did the movements together and after about 30 seconds Rachel peeked at me. We continued a little longer and then Rachel stopped. She said she could see the connection between movement and feeling when she watched me, but, in herself, she felt no such connection.

Her head roll was awkward, the muscles around her neck and shoulders were tight. But although Rachel seemed uncomfortable, she said she liked the new challenge and wanted to do more. She said she was especially happy to move alongside of me and this, in and of itself, held special significance. The goal of uniting mind and body, of endowing her movements with feeling, was still remote.

Rachel did become excited about starting to move in the sessions and began to bring in her favorite "feeling music." She reported that The Kids were proud of themselves. Finally they were moving. It didn't seem to matter what movement we chose as long as it was simple and to music that was meaningful to Rachel. When she spoke of the movement, it was in terms of how it felt to move with me. "The Kids like dancing with you. Do you like dancing with them?" She was always surprised to learn how much I enjoyed moving and doing creative activities with her. As a child she had yearned for experiences like these with her mother. But, as an adult, she recognized that her mother could not promote this kind of freedom perhaps because she, herself, had never been allowed this experience.

It became clear that The Kids could not be expected to find their own way. In the area of expressive movement, The Kids were still very young. They needed and demanded interaction. Any attempts to help Rachel to move alone were met with, "I don't know what to do" but at home Rachel had begun to play music and move. About this experience she said "all I do is sway." When I asked her if she enjoyed swaying she said "yes." She remembered that as a child she had a hard time standing without moving and often swayed back and forth. Her mother made fun of her and said, "Can't you ever just stand still?" Rachel was embarrassed about the swaying but did not have control over this partially unconscious act. Rocking back and forth from one leg to the other is often a movement one does to calm oneself. It is like the rocking of a baby and may, in fact, indicate that the rocker is unwittingly nurturing a younger part of the self, as was probably the case for Rachel.

Because it was the one movement with which Rachel was comfortable, we spent a good deal of time swaying to music. Doing so gave Rachel pleasure but she also wanted to extend her movement repertoire.

I did not expect Rachel to be able to engage in movement on her own, solely from internal prompting. Her parents had inhibited her childlike spontaneity and had placed severe restrictions on all expression of feeling. The body had become linked in Rachel's mind with shame and humiliation. In order for Rachel to unlock the physical restraints her fears placed on The Kids, she needed a role model and guide to whom she could safely attach while she rid herself of the physically paralyzing influence of her parents.

The question remained. How could Rachel learn to express herself with her body? The answer became clearer. We needed to start at The Kids' level of physical development. Rachel had adapted to childhood dilemmas by separating her intellectual, vocational, and academic strivings from painful childhood emotions. Her emotions had been repressed. They had never found physical expression. It was as if she needed to restrain her body in order to restrain her feelings. Therefore, even though The Kids matured on many levels, their physical expressivity lagged behind. Although Rachel was no longer completely dependent on me to help her formulate her thoughts and feelings, she was dependent on me to express herself in movement.

I concluded that Rachel needed to see and imitate movement in the same way that an infant sees and imitates. With this in mind I invited Rachel to mirror my movements. Mirroring seemed to have a freeing effect on her, not unlike the way a child learns to verbalize through imitation. Rachel began to learn the vocabulary of movement. All language, be it the language of art, dance, or words, provides another form through which children can express themselves. But to acquire this new form, they have to start first with the rudiments—a single word, a movement, a shape or color.

In the beginning, The Kids seemed satisfied to explore new movement solely through mirroring. There was, however, an ingredient missing. The movements lacked a motivational spark that would bring them more fully alive. It was important to find a way to elicit the essence of The Kids through movement. Mirroring, creativity, and Rachel's exceptional ability to visualize all waited to be brought out through spontaneous dance and movement.

The Kids found a solution. Rachel brought in the music from "Beauty and the Beast" and suggested we dance to it. She chose her favorite song and asked me if I would move with her. We began by swaying back and forth together while standing side by side. Rachel was a little embarrassed and didn't look at me. I encouraged some expansion of the swaying movement by suggesting that she sway in different directions (side to side, front and back, up and down). When the song ended, the next piece was the background music for a scene in which the Beast ran after Beauty to bring her back to his castle. In this scene the Beast is attacked by wolves and Beauty comes to his rescue, after which he is transformed by Beauty's love into the handsome Prince. As the music played Rachel narrated the story while I found dance movements to portray and embellish Rachel's words. Following my lead, Rachel became animated and joined in. Together we danced the story of "Beauty and the Beast."

At its heart, "Beauty and the Beast" is the story of the transformation of the self through love, and Rachel understood its message very well. The story had always moved The Kids deeply.

Rachel had found a vehicle for helping herself to integrate form and feeling, mind and body, and Rachel and The Kids. She left a joyous message on my answering machine that night, "The Kids were happy all day. They can't stop talking about dancing. They had so much fun and can't wait to dance with you again!"

One Year Later—In Rachel's Own Words

I recently had a job interview, the first one in almost 12 years. It was with a prestigious company that would be a good fit for me and believe it or not, I networked to get it. Much to my surprise, the interview went well and I got a lot of positive feedback. More important than the interview itself, I caught a glimpse of some of the positive changes in me. The discussion was a wonderful blend of Nameless and FJ—an engaging, personable Nameless and a knowledgeable, determined FJ. We were focused, articulate, and able to make eye contact with the interviewer. We covered most of the important points and if we missed any or wanted to clarify further, brought the conversation back to enable us to do so. Afterwards, I marveled at all the changes in me.

There is one story that summarizes how I view my personal growth over the last several years. It is from the story of Sybil (Schreiber, 1984):

> There was once a mother ant and her daughter. They lived in an ant hill—a comfortable home—but the location wasn't suitable. It was noisy and when the wind blew, some of the rooftop went with it. The ants decided that it was time to move their ant hill to the other side of town. Both were aghast when they thought of the task ahead—moving the ant hill one grain of sand at a time from one side of town to the other. They were determined, though, and started the job. It took many years; there was much sweat and tears but there were also joyful moments that came from working together and sharing the burden. Finally, the ant hill was moved and the ants were jubilant. The mother ant and her daughter hugged each other and the mother said, "Isn't it amazing what two ants can do when they work together!"

There are moments, similar to the job interview, when I can see how much the kids and I have grown. I sit back, astounded, and think, isn't it amazing what we have done in our work together!

Postscript

As of this writing, Rachel and I continue to meet three times a week and we have phone sessions on the days she does not come to the office. She no longer suffers from depression or disabling anxiety. The frequent stomach problems and insomnia that she initially presented are all but gone. Occasionally she complains of a stubborn headache. The problems she had concentrating at work have also disappeared.

Concerning Rachel's career, she remained at the same corporation and advanced to vice-president. She also got the position she interviewed for in 1995 and is doing well with her new and ever-increasing responsibilities. The fear of flying that had prevented her from traveling and had made business trips a nightmare has abated.

Of major concern at this time is that Rachel experiences herself as abnormally high strung and as, at times, fiercely rageful at small provocation. She notes, "I would like to be a nicer, more accepting person but I'm not there yet. I still have a long way to go." Now that the constraints on Rachel have been lifted and she is more in touch with her anger and aggression, she wonders if she is capable of compassion for others. The very fact that she asks this question and expresses a genuine concern points strongly in the direction of a positive answer.

Rachel is also concerned that she currently prefers her own company to the company of others. She reports feeling confined and controlled when she is with others, overdefined by their expectations and needs, but is happy in her own company.

She describes many moments, especially on weekends and holidays, of complete joy, "when I push up the windows in my sparkling clean apartment, put on my favorite classical music, take out a cook book and all of my wonderful fruits, vegetables, and cooking utensils and I feel completely free and at peace." Even though she usually prefers being alone, Rachel does have friends who are important to her. She has also begun to form a meaningful relationship with her parents.

Rachel continues to experience herself as a composite of different selves, but not with the same anguish or severity of her earlier days. The Kids have grown significantly and their demands on her have diminished. They are now a happier, more integrated unit. The end goal is not for her to give up her multiplicity but rather for her to continue to openly express all of her thoughts and feelings and for her to continue maturing into her own person—free of anger and hurt from the past and free to become, in effect, *one happy family who have learned to live together.*

2

Dancing beyond Trauma:
Women Survivors of Sexual Abuse

Bonnie Bernstein

When a young girl or woman is sexually violated, she often experiences a trauma to every aspect of her being. As her body has been invaded, all normal physical and emotional boundaries have been disregarded. The combined psychological and physical impact of her experience may leave her with scars that alter her relationship to her body and to her world forever. Because dance therapy emphasizes the complex interaction of the psyche and the body, it provides an invaluable form of treatment for such women. Presented here is a particular dance therapy orientation that has evolved from years of both individual and group dance therapy with women survivors of sexual trauma.

Adult sexual trauma survivors have diverse histories. They include women who have been raped as adults or as children as well as those who have been victimized by incest, childhood molestation, date rape, war rape, or ritual abuse. Their stories are often shocking and horrific. The rape survivor has usually experienced real violence, often including a threat to her life. The incest survivor has in addition experienced psychological abuse, manipulation, and a breach of familial love and trust. All survivors are left with emotional scars, among them injured self-concept, guilt, shame, and depression. Many survivors also experience relationship difficulties or sexual dysfunction. Moreover, a survivor may be left with an injured relationship to her body. This includes body image, movement style, physical expression, and interaction between her feelings and life actions.

Effective verbal therapy for the survivor emphasizes improving self-concept and working through painful memories. Treatment frequently includes improving relationship skills and changing the dissatisfying life-styles that may have evolved (Gil, 1988). In addition dance therapy emphasizes improving the survivor's relationship to her body. Through movement she is helped to recognize and change the ways she uses, abuses, or inhibits her body. In dance therapy the body becomes at once the vehicle for change and the focus of change, so that the client can begin to reclaim her body as an ally in her struggle toward health.

Blanche Evan's Methods

The work described in this chapter is based on the theory and methods of Blanche Evan (Benov, 1991; Levy, 1988; Rifkin-Gainer, Bernstein, & Melson, 1984). The Evan approach emphasizes restoring the client to her natural potential for expressive movement and "re-educating the body to a state wherein movement responses function" (Evan, 1951, p. 88). It also mobilizes the dynamic interaction between the psyche and the body. Toward this end the work includes dance education and movement rehabilitation in addition to emphasis on in-depth exploration of feelings and insight-oriented improvisation. The Evan method serves as primary, rather than adjunctive treatment, and is appropriate for clients who possess the ego strength to tolerate in-depth self-examination. The following section will provide a brief explanation of Blanche Evan's terms that are used by the author to describe session sequences and interventions.

Psycho-physical refers to an experience that occurs concurrently on psychological and physical levels and describes the complex impact that the body has on the psyche, and that the psyche has on the body. A fundamental concept to the Evan's method, *psycho-physical* implies that all human experience including emotional response, memory, and thoughts contain kinesthetic components. Body movement is a direct outlet for the psyche, thus, through dance, the *psycho-physical* realm can be fully expressed and explored to stimulate insight and mobilize therapeutic change. "To experience *psycho-physical* unity is a basic need" (Evan, 1949, p. 54).

Mobilization refers to sequences of directives that are formulated to increase body awareness and broaden movement vocabulary through the exploration of the elements of dance, that is, rhythm, space, intensity, body movement, and content. "A goal is to open up the client's body without taking away defenses. Moving, expanding, and discovering the body without pointing it to content" (Evan, 1978, personal communication). Three examples of *mobilizations* are: (1) a directive emphasizing body structure, such as exploring the range of movement of the spine; (2) a directive expanding the use of dance elements, such as gradually varying tempo from very fast to very slow; and (3) a directive that encourages experimenting with new movement dynamics, such as to explore leaping, sliding, lunging, and exploding.

Improvisation refers to the Evan method of insight-oriented dance, characterized by free association in movement and guided by psychological, physical, or *psycho-physical* themes. "Improvisation is dependent on an over-all state of receptivity which is replaced with identification with your theme. At the point of action, it is the summation of your past and present. It is also the arbiter between reality and fantasy" (Evan, 1950, p. 80). *Improvisation* gives physical form to psychological experiences and Evan states: "Honest *improvisation* is a direct route to the unconscious" (Benov, 1991, p. 192). In this work, content-evoking themes are suggested by the therapist in response to a client's verbal and/or movement communications. Four examples of improvisation techniques, as defined by Evan, are *"externalizing," "enacting," "physicalizing,"* and *"rehearsing."* In *externalizing* the client might "dance out" a dream, fantasy, or physical memory. In *enacting*, the client recreates a significant life experience, perhaps her assault, and while dancing, she may embellish the life *enactment* with movement derived from previously unexpressed feelings. *Physicalizing* involves putting into movement an idea, a memory, or a feeling that has been previously stored in a cognitive realm. *Rehearsing* involves an *improvisation* in which alternative responses are created and practiced in order to prepare for changes in behavior outside of the therapy session.

Functional techniques ™ refers to a movement-education approach developed by Blanche Evan to focus on body mechanics. It includes a series of systematic exercise progressions and movement sequences to increase strength, flexibility, and resiliency. In the Evan method, rehabilitating the body is intrinsic to the restoration of psycho-physical health. Through this work the client is helped to release "non-functional" tensions, modify movement habits, and restore the natural abilities of the body. *"Functional technique* is not an accessory, but an integral ingredient within the whole therapy process" (Evan, 1979, Personal Communication).

Ethnic dance, which enhances the therapy process, includes resources of multi-cultural dance and music, such as the creation of dances inspired by international music, the inclusion of therapeutic dance rituals based on those from other cultures, and the utilization of ethnic movements and dances to evoke specific emotional content.

Creative dance, as taught in the method of Blanche Evan, provides experiences that can stimulate the client's often limited or inhibited use of imagination, fantasy, and imagery. The dancing themes such as the violence of a storm, the aggression of a wild animal, or the building intensity of waves, may enable a client to express a range of feelings and body states, without direct focus on painful issues. Evan developed a unique style of using *creative dance* as a bridge to insight-oriented improvisation (Benov, 1991).

Language and vocalization are actively utilized in Blanche Evan's methods. Liberating the voice in emotive expression is encouraged. To "actionize words" (Evan, 1979, Personal Communication) is to *improvise* on a specific verbal statement, so as to elicit meaningful content. A client might, for example, "actionize" the statement "I feel tormented" by dancing her own experience of torment in movements of twisting tension and perseveration. In a more usual use of verbalization, discussion among group members can create peer support and articulate important links between the client's dance experiences and her life.

Homework is encouraged in the Evan method. From homework the client learns how to bring new insights and new movement skills into actions taken between therapy sessions. "The client needs to know that work is not done in session, but during the week, and clarified in session" (Evan, 1980, Personal Communication). Homework, developed out of session material, helps to connect therapy to life outside of therapy and encourages autonomy while promoting life-style change. Examples of homework include noticing one's movements while speaking to a boss or improvising with assertive movements before visiting family members.

In sum, Evan's theories and methods serve as a rich foundation for work with sexual-assault survivors. Evan states "Experiencing the physical equivalent of the psyche in body action is a universal basic need which the dance is abundantly qualified to fill" (cited in Benov, 1991, p. 57). As the survivor is exposed to the world of movement she is provided with invaluable tools for healing.

Choreography of a Dance Therapy Session for Survivors: The Therapist–Client Dynamic

From the onset of treatment, the therapist's steadfast belief in the client's ability to work through her trauma sets the stage for a relationship that is both supportive and encouraging of growth and change. Each session emphasizes the survivor's physical autonomy and unique pathway toward health. This is particularly evident in a style of therapist–client interaction that is characteristic of the Blanche Evan Method. Poised on the sidelines, the therapist watches with acute concentration and empathy in order to direct and respond to her client. The therapist intentionally refrains from demonstrating movements or improvising with the client except in carefully chosen instances. This therapist–client dynamic encourages the survivor toward independence and toward the discovery of her personal style of using the elements of dance and psychophysical expression. The author has developed a format of group dance therapy that incorporates this emphasis on the client's autonomy, and at the same time mobilizes the therapeutic assets of group interaction.

The following excerpts from group and individual therapy sessions will highlight themes that frequently arise for the survivor: shame, guilt, dissociation, dysfunctional sexuality, dissatisfying interpersonal relationships, developmental issues, and finally, trauma resolution. Case examples illustrate the theoretical and clinical significance of specific dance therapy interventions.

Dancing Past Shame

A survivor may enter therapy with symptoms of shame but not relate this shame to her sexual trauma. She may have an aversion to body parts or bodily functions, suffer from eating disorders, protect her body with unflattering attire, or suffer from poor social skills and depression. Shame produces an overall state of inhibition that blocks self-expression, movement freedom, and spontaneity. One client said, "I felt that if I got fat enough no one would see me. When I became obese, I was able to mask the shame I felt about my incest with the shame I felt about my weight." The following session describes dance therapy interventions used to help a group of survivors work through shame.

The group session, which was attended by six female incest survivors, began with a directive to loosen arm and leg joints and explore a range of movements in a variety of directions in space. I asked the women to explore "stepping out in new ways" on different levels, using asymmetrical movement to the front, side, diagonal, and backward. Their inhibitions decreased as they experimented with new uses of space and afterwards I asked each group member to describe how she might be stepping out in new ways in her life. One woman spoke of letting a neighbor into her home. She was struck by how new this behavior was, given how she usually kept everyone out. She connected her habit to the shame and secrecy that surrounded the home of her family of origin. The group talked of their common experiences of hiding while growing up, of shame related to sexual assault and other painful memories: an embarrassing alcoholic mother, a messy, chaotic house, and an exhibitionist stepfather.

To deepen the process of identifying the psycho-physical impact of the past I encouraged the group to generate memories of their own childhood bodies and to physicalize positions and movements that reflected their corresponding feelings. The explorations revealed movements of tension, holding, hiding, provocative showing off, sneaking, and withdrawing. To expand on this theme, I suggested that each woman recreate and physicalize a significant experience that evoked shame, or explore how this feeling manifested itself in their adult bodies. One woman portrayed the bodies of both her parents in endless bickering. Her dance evolved into movements of hiding and withdrawal, an expression of the self denigration she felt after she was abused by her father. Another improvised frustration and powerlessness at her inability to protect her mother from her stepfather's beatings. A third woman scurried in circular motions from one end of the room to the other, expressing the overwhelming disorganization she experienced in the past and in the present. After their concurrent dances, the group again talked about their feelings of shame and alienation. They recounted that, as children, they had felt evil or dirty and each had desperately tried to hide from their peers both their dysfunctional families and her incest secrets.

The initial directive in the first phase of the session exemplifies how movement is a bridge to content-laden themes. As the survivor remembers her history with her body, she begins to explore her kinesthetic memories and previously unexpressed emotional responses through insight-oriented improvisation.

To further explore the content of the dances, I guided the group toward additional dances. The woman who expressed guilt for not protecting her mother was asked, how old she was at the time of the memory. She said "5." To help her depict her childhood size as it had compared to her stepfather's, a taller group member stood on a chair to characterize the large, wide body. Using the spatial elements of size and level, she recognized her long-held distortion of reality. The 5-year-old child's small stature and powerlessness were painfully obvious to the group. As a result of this enactment, she was able to redirect the blame from herself to her stepfather.

The next phase of this session suggests how physical and emotional power can be enhanced through the use of ethnic music and dance. To the sounds of Creole drums, I encouraged the group to create a movement ritual. I suggested they dance to the phrase "Move the shame out of your bodies." The movements that evolved were, at first, individual actions of flinging, shaking, and rubbing off of body surfaces. The group then added their own verbalizations: "I was only 5. I couldn't protect my mother!" and "Leave her alone!" Group chanting of one person's words helped to affirm everyone. For some, not yet able to assert their own anger, the experience of using their voices to help another assists in building their own self-confidence. In Evan's words: "Making sounds means I exist—I can be heard" (Evan, 1976, Personal Communication).

Dissociation and Dancing Toward Integration

Dissociative disorder refers to "a disturbance or alteration in the normally integrative functions of identity, memory or consciousness" (American Psychiatric Association, 1987, p. 269). Aspects of this disorder include (a) depersonalization disorder, in which the customary feeling of one's own reality is replaced by a feeling of unreality; (b) psychogenic amnesia and psychogenic fugue, in which the disturbance occurs primarily in memory and important events or specific time periods cannot be recalled; and (c) multiple personality disorder, in which the disturbance occurs primarily in identity. The individual's customary identity is temporarily forgotten, and a new identity may be assumed or imposed. The following discussion is limited to the first two types of dissociation, as treatment of multiple personality disorder is beyond the scope of this chapter.

During a sexual trauma, dissociation serves as an adaptive survival strategy. As the body is being violated, the survivor seeks to preserve the integrity of her personality by "splitting off" from her body (Gil, 1988). When the sexual intrusion abates, the survivor's defense often persists, with a variety of physical symptoms such as deadness or numbness of her body, partial amnesia, states described as "out of my skin" or "spaced out," and sensations of unreality. One client said, "I was being repeatedly raped by a large man, I felt like I was going to die. I focussed on the quietness around me and felt numb. Four years later I still feel numb." Many such survivors are high functioning and have developed techniques to mask their symptoms. Those who associate often experience life from a witness perspective, however (Schilder, 1950), and when confronted with issues of authority or intimacy may retreat in their minds to what they describe as another place, away from their bodies. The therapist may be able to detect dissociation, for example, only through a slight turning of the eyes or a less-focused stare. Such an individual often feels uncomfortable and out of control, even though her flight may be to the safety of a fantasy world.

Treatment for dissociation requires several stages of intervention. First, the therapist must help the survivor decrease her shame and come to terms with secrets regarding the dissociation. Many survivors are relieved to have this private experience witnessed, identified, and defined. A second stage, which is particularly accessible through dance therapy, involves exploring the survivor's images and symbols. Improvisations that articulate the dissociative process can stimulate the survivor's insight into the strategies she has developed. Memories not available through ordinary channels may be evoked when the client is dancing aspects of her altered states. Through psycho-physical explorations she may uncover what occurred during her initial body–mind split. A third stage is to help the client develop skills and strategies for controlling her flights from reality. The following session with Martha, illustrates work with dissociation.

Martha said, "I would focus on the ceiling while my stepfather molested me. I floated upward to a land where I was safe...I would be a princess where everyone was kind to me. I imagined sitting in my grandmother's lap. I felt warm and safe."

Martha's language provides clues to her internal experience. For example, her dissociative defense is illustrated in her intense "focus on the ceiling" and in her image of "floating upward" away from herself. Her language also depicts movement qualities, those of intensity and floating. The elements of movement revealed by language represent important aspects of the self. Martha's dances expressing "where she went" during her flights and "how she got there" enabled her to recall what she had repressed.

When I directed Martha to improvise on the "floating upward" image, she raised and lowered her arms in circular and airy motions, while her eyes stayed fixed upward on the wall. She scraped the wall as if trying to move into it, then hid her eyes with her hands and, in rigid tension and distress, grabbed a scarf to cover her face. Because her eyes seemed to be central in her dance, I asked her, "What do you see? What do you not want to see?" Martha danced herself as a distorted freak. She added shrill yells and grunts as expressions of ugliness and finally with large, forceful punching movements she screamed, "Get away from me!"

After her dance, Martha said "My lifeline during my abuse was my fixation on the wall. Somehow if I didn't see him (stepfather) I could imagine this was not happening to me. I was somewhere else, and I still go there." She was surprised to discover that her flight was not primarily from her stepfather but rather from her own feelings of self-disgust. Martha connected the self-hate in her dance to feelings she kept secret in her adult life, and also connected the childhood strategy of eye contact to her adult dissociation. She said, "I still find safety in floating above my feelings and away from direct communication with people."

In later sessions, Martha improvised on the interactions between the princess, the grandmother, and the child. In time she began to observe the abused little girl below her while she floated above and felt empathy for the abandoned part of her self. She eventually created tender dances of protection using the three characters in her imagery. As these characters were able to inter-act and unify, she experienced all of them as aspects of her self and her need for dissociative defenses decreased.

Defining Body Boundaries

"Body image" is a term that "refers to the body as a psychological experience and focuses on the individual's feelings and attitudes toward his own body" (Fisher, 1968, p. x). Body boundaries involve the "demarcation line between one's own body and that which is outside one's body" (Fisher & Cleveland, 1968, p. 52). Body boundaries are shaped by the past and become "a basis of operation" for dealing with the world (Fisher & Cleveland, 1968, p. 56). Sexual-trauma survivors often come to therapy with disrupted physical as well as emotional boundaries (Blume, 1991). Such disruption manifests not only in the survivor's self-concept but also in her relationships to others. She may have difficulty establishing limits, articulating opinions, or approaching intimacy. Improvisation augmented by movement education helps the survivor develop spatial clarity, control, and autonomy. The following illustrates how dance ther-apy interventions encourage greater definition of body boundaries.

Prior to this session, as homework each group member had made a body-image drawing accompanied by written explanations of both positive and neg-ative associations to body parts. We began with mobilization directives that encouraged full movement of the area each woman identified with positive feel-ings. Then I asked everyone to choose a partner who could help her focus on a negatively associated area. During these interactions the women experienced a nonthreatening introduction to movements of their most uncomfortable body areas. They also experienced a challenge to their negative and inhibited move-ment patterns and the accompanying associations. The movements evolved into a group dance of work actions such as pounding with a mortar and pes-tle, cutting wheat with a scythe, and stomping grapes.

I then directed the group to explore a new range of movement facili-tated by the terms bend, reach, wiggle, and dart. In addition, qualities such as wild, explosive, gentle, rigid, and strong were also suggested. Such movement challenges increase body awareness, enliven numbed areas, and help the sur-vivor experience her physical boundaries.

To enhance boundary definition I introduced Functional Technique sequences that focused on exercise to strengthen the spine and torso: undula-tions of the spine that articulated movement of individual vertebrae, rotations of the spine through different planes, and unified spinal action with the limbs.

We then broadened the exercises to the alignment of the head, neck, shoulder, and torso. Drawing from ethnic movement, I offered an image of a proud African woman strolling gracefully with a basket on her head. In response to the image, the group members lengthened their spines further. This phase of the group ended with a liberating dance to African drum music.

Next, with reference to the body-image drawings, I suggested that the group improvise to the phrase, "my body boundaries." One woman began with her sensation of being "marsh-like" and gradually made the transition to more boundary-defined movements. This stimulated her awareness of the struggle she was having to maintain healthy boundaries within her marriage. Another woman who often felt "invisible" used her strengthened spinal movements to "take command." A third woman enacted her alcoholic mother's movements and realized that she had adopted many of her mother's mannerisms. Through improvisation, she discovered that her identification with her mother existed on a deep physical level. In her own body she experienced her mother's vulnerability. This insight led to future dances that helped her to individuate from her mother.

Dancing Past Guilt

The rape survivor may come to treatment with feelings of guilt and responsibility about having been attacked (Brownmiller, 1975). The incest survivor, plagued by the aftermath of chronic abuse, may believe that the sexual invasion was brought on by her own actions (Blume, 1991). One woman said, "If only I had run away when he said he had the knife, I might have prevented my rape." Another said, "My stepfather called me a sexy slut, and said it was the way I moved that provoked him." In both cases, a reexamination of false assumptions helped to relieve guilt and self-condemnation.

Residues of guilt are tenaciously retained in the survivor's body and may contribute to sexual inhibition, promiscuity, tension, inability to experience pleasure, and fear of risk taking. Guilt may also manifest in the survivor's inability to trust her own choices and in an urgent need to remain in control. One approach is to focus on specific experiences that led to the guilty feelings. Another, as in the following session, is to focus on the survivor's body, and to develop dance experiences that free the survivor from the physical restrictions that represent the guilt.

In the first phase of this particular session, group members talked about how they inhibited themselves in their lives. Over and over guilt was identified as the root of the self-restricting behaviors and of decreasing self-trust. The discussion of guilt led to a focus on "letting go" physically. We began with mobilization directives. A series of full-bodied swing progressions were used to release muscular tension, to feel the spontaneity associated with building momentum, and to invigorate numbed body areas. Frequently the survivor of sexual abuse numbs and constricts feelings and actions within the body. These symptoms are often routed in unconscious associations and guilt. Although the group members showed new freedom of movement in their dances, a consistent lack of resiliency in their knees and legs restricted full hip and pelvic action. Functional technique exercises for the knees and legs were introduced to encourage both loosening and strengthening. Releasing physical restrictions enables the expression of qualities such as assertion and sensuality, which guilt may have inhibited. The group ended with a dance to Middle Eastern music, which integrated resilient knee action with full hip and pelvic movement. These movements encouraged locomotion through space without inhibition.

In the next phase of the session, I offered a creative dance directive in which each survivor was encouraged to select an image from nature to stimulate a dance of release and "letting go." In doing so they increased their expressive freedom without having to confront the content of their inhibitions.

The next task was to bridge the group's creative dance experience to their psycho-physical manifestations of guilt. Again the group improvised themes of "letting go" and resiliency. One person let go of "beating herself up" with guilt. Her initial inward focus turned outward into a dance of powerful rage. Another woman concentrated on the ways guilt related to her tendency to dissociate. She used the resilient and stabilizing knee-bending exercises from earlier in the session in an effort to prevent her tendency to "leave her body." A third woman who danced to explore her sexuality, expressed the flurry of thoughts that distracted her from being emotionally present with her husband during lovemaking. As she worked on releasing her spine and thigh muscles, she danced images of "letting go" sexually. In the closing portion of the session, I encouraged each group member to create a poem for her images. Each recitation was accompanied by flute music and followed by individual improvisations.

This session demonstrates the interplay of several dance therapy interventions. Mobilization and Functional Technique altered habitual and constricted movement patterns. Creative dance stimulated expression and imagination while broadening dance skills. Improvisation helped explore how guilt restricted personal freedom. Change in movement itself can bring about a change in attitude that, in turn, can liberate the survivor. The primary focus of this session was on the body and the issue of "letting go," rather then on the origins or specific content of guilt.

Bridging Gaps in Development

Emotional damage to the survivor results not only from the sexual crime, but from the ongoing family dynamic that allows the incest to occur (Herman, 1981). Parents who are alcoholic, violent, co-dependent, or sociopathic shape the incest victim's view of the world. Many survivors grow up in constant fear and, as adults, experience grief over lost childhood. Thus, dance therapy must include a focus on the disruption of normal development. She may require work in areas of communication, assertiveness, and conflict resolution. The survivor's body image must be extricated from enmeshment with her dysfunctional family and transformed to one of increased psycho-physical strength and autonomy.

Many incest survivors are unable to play, laugh, or enjoy life. Dance therapy provides these normal childhood experiences, through the use of play themes and childhood imagery. Directives to generate childlike movements that are gawky, unpredictable, or asymmetrical often shake the survivor out of rigid movement patterns. Experiments in spontaneity can encourage playfulness in adult life.

Props such as percussion instruments, costumes, children's music, and drum recordings all stimulate play themes. Photographs, paintings, poetry or literature depicting children and adults in playful abandon can evoke freeing imagery. Folk and ethnic dance provide another vehicle for freeing movement. In one session the group was taught a seal dance from Tierra del Fuego (grunts and scratching included), a leaping butterfly dance from Japan, and a yelling, kicking-out dance from Nigeria. With these dances, the group experienced liberating movement, laughter, and camaraderie in play.

Another developmental need is to instill a positive attitude toward the self. Here the therapist's positive regard and belief in the survivor's strengths is significant. To improve self-concept, the sessions include experiences of affirmation. Members demonstrate ways they have acted in their own behalf; they form a "circle of shared compliments," or they demonstrate movements that express their strengths. A positive vision of the future can be stimulated through dancing hopes and dreams.

Dances of Power: A Foundation for Healthier Relationships

It is not unusual for the survivor to experience herself as a victim. Her memories of powerlessness, fear, and loss of control damage her capacity to form healthy relationships. The survivor must learn to communicate her needs and feelings in order to experience equality and intimacy.

Feeling ineffectual has significant psycho-physical components. A survivor, forced into silence by her perpetrator, must regain her voice. A survivor who has protected herself by confining her movements must learn to reclaim a space in the world. When a survivor identifies with images of power and assertion she begins to build a sense of strength and control. Only by altering her self-image can she leave behind the victim stance. The following focuses on dance therapy interventions that contribute to feeling effective.

I began with the suggestion that each group member describe her physical needs with a spontaneous "moving-talking body sculpture." In response to the group's spontaneous facial expression, I suggested they add sounds and whole-body movements. This in turn led to a "body-sounds" dance, followed by a powerful group chant. To further activate their voices, I suggested they create gibberish arguments with partners. A playful argument in gibberish is not as intimidating as an actual argument, but it does exercise the individual's assertive affect, and permits a range of vocal expressions.

Exhilarated by their ability to use their voices in powerful sound, the women began to talk about their memories of powerlessness. They said, "I can feel my arms now. Usually my arms and shoulders don't belong to me. They were too weak to fight back." "I had no legs. They usually feel numb and lifeless." To focus on building muscular strength in the body areas the group experienced as weak, I introduced a Functional Technique directive that included leg lifts for abdominal muscles and thighs; scapula isolations to strengthen arms; and a progression of body arcs to stretch, strengthen, and unify the arms, torso, and legs. This movement education provided not only sensations of power and control but actually increased body strength. According to Schilder (1950), body image is shaped through movement and for the survivor, healthy movement experiences contribute to reshaping negative body images.

Next the group spontaneously devised dances that helped them feel more assertive. The women took turns using both movement and words to make strong statements to someone in their lives: "I insist that you listen to me when I tell you this!" "I am a worthwhile person and deserve to be treated with respect!" "You cannot touch me again!"

In the closing phase, the group identified and physicalized ways in which each person had contributed to her own survival during the assault. Finally the group examined ways to use their survival strengths in their current relationships.

Dancing Memories: Trauma Resolution

Many survivors suffer from posttraumatic stress disorder, which is defined as the development of particular symptoms as the result of an event that is outside the range of usual experience (American Psychiatric Association, 1994). Characteristic symptoms included repeated reexperience of the traumatic event, avoidance of stimuli associated with the event, numbing of general responsiveness, or state of increased arousal. Treatment includes confronting memories and integrating cognitive, affective, and physiologic responses (Gil, 1988).

Catharsis through dance releases unexpressed feeling and memories and is an important part of trauma resolution. The following highlights the effectiveness of tracking memories that emerge through movement.

Janet was a soft-spoken young woman who felt unusual tightness in her throat; she had worked on releasing her voice in previous sessions. She began a dance that intensified the constriction and followed her associations to this tightness. She shifted from standing to lying on the floor and began to remember and reenact a childhood memory in which her father forced her to perform fellatio. This invasion had not only made it impossible for her to scream, but also restricted her ability to breathe. She had feared she would die of suffocation as she silently waited for him to ejaculate. I encouraged Janet to use her voice and breath to express the feelings and the sounds inhibited in the past. She gave liberating yells and deep grunts of disgust; she externalized her rage with animal-like movements and sounds. She stomped her feet with power, symbolically threw her father away from her, and stood her ground on solid legs.

By following her associations, Janet experienced catharsis. The psychophysical release freed her to view her past from a changed body state and, thus, a different perspective. Janet retrieved buried memories and recaptured her voice, strength, and verticality. The experience of standing her ground eventually led her to confront her father.

Movement Styles and Post-traumatic Defenses

Attention to each dance element: rhythm, space, dynamics, body movement, and content can be key in trauma resolution. The survivor's daily use or avoidance of particular dance elements can be indicative of a limited movement range shaped by posttraumatic avoidance.

Joan, a rape survivor, characteristically moved at a slow tempo. This lethargy and diminished intensity included inhibition of joyous excitement, muted sexual passion, and inability to express anger. She recognized an aversion to quick or intense movement, but was clueless as to why. Through many sessions Joan experimented with varying her tempo. Using photographs from her youth, she worked to capture energetic movement. She danced to the crescendo and diminuendo of a gong.

In a pivotal improvisation I asked Joan to move as her rapist had moved. In this dance she began to uncover both the terror of her rape experience and the origins of her diminished tempo. By leaving her victim role she liberated intensity in her own body and experienced the power of her attacker. When Joan completed her dance, she was able to move with increased tempo and intensity. She clarified that her fear of rageful violence from her rapist had robbed her of her freedom of movement.

Joan's posttraumatic stress was manifested in her avoidance of quick tempo and intensity. Posttraumatic stress may similarly inhibit a survivor's use of space, levels, directionality, or areas of the body. Thus trauma resolution can be aided by uncovering origins of movement styles and focusing on recapturing full range of motion.

Rehearsals and Reenactments

The following focuses on another element of trauma resolution: rehearsal for confrontation. For many survivors, rage turns inward into self-destructive behavior or depression. In the next session, an incest survivor is able to confront her perpetrator, turning the rage outward.

Mindy, who had been sexually molested by her father from age 7 to 11, suffered from chronic depression. Faced with her father's deteriorating health, she was presented with a last opportunity to communicate her feelings to him. In previous sessions, dance improvisations had uncovered ambivalence. She danced a childlike expression of longing for her daddy's love and acceptance, together with her physical discomfort and terror when he slipped into her room at night. She had enacted a dreaded memory of pretending to be asleep as he abused her; and she had unleashed unexpressed anger at him for stripping her of her innocence. Mindy had also externalized her chronic depression through dance.

Mindy prepared for the visit with her father by rehearsing. This provided her opportunities to release feelings that might later be inhibited when she confronted her father. Mindy both moved and verbalized all her feelings for her father. I encouraged her not to censor anything and assured her that she could later choose what to communicate and what to withhold. In one session, group members helped her to express accusations and rage. Her words were affirmed by the group's supporting voices and movements. She also practiced a dialogue with another group member, who responded to her statements with the counter-attacks she anticipated from her father: "You wanted it! You provoked it! You're crazy, it didn't happen!" Supported by the group, Mindy rehearsed self-validating responses.

Mindy's actual confrontation with her father was, in fact, much less eventful than her preparation. Although his condition severely limited his comprehension, the process of preparation and the opportunity to follow though changed Mindy. The lasting impact was a lifting of the depression and a sense of deep satisfaction.

The final example of trauma-resolution work focuses on the value of cognitive education augmented by physicalization. The survivor often benefits from learning that her denial, self-blame, depression, and anger are all commonly experienced post-rape responses. It also helps her to understand that she "did the best she could" during the assault. This learning has more lasting impact when it is experienced physically as well as verbally.

Dana, a rape survivor, was tormented by the idea that she could have somehow prevented her assault. She repeatedly fantasized alternative actions she might have taken. I encouraged her to dance an enactment of the rape and to include the changes she imagined. As she danced. she discovered that if she had tried to fight back, the rapist's knife might have injured her more seriously. After this, Dana understood that her intuitive actions had actually helped her to survive.

Reclaiming Sexuality

Disruptions in sexuality are a common scar following sexual trauma. Symptoms include disturbance of desire, inability to achieve orgasm, inhibition or even dissociation sparked by intimacy, trauma flashbacks, and a variety of sexual aversions and fears (Blume, 1991).

In a sexuality workshop for survivors, *creative dance* opened doors to liberating sexual function. First I asked the group to list words that implied sensuality: "Slinky, shaking, undulating, smooth, daring, flowing, and rhythmic." They then danced their responses to each word. The dances stimulated new movement qualities that evoked associations to sensuality. Then I asked the group to dance an image from literature or a painting that captured some aspect of womanliness they admired. The dances included movements of power, solidity, strength, sensuality, nurturing, and aggression.

Sexuality is often inhibited by the unconscious linking of body sensations with traumatic memories. Through dance the physicality of sex can be separated from the violence of sexual assault, the feeling of letting go separated from the act of giving in, being open separated from being exposed. Passion can be distinguished from aggression, self-protection from inhibition, and healthful control of one's body from control that squelches sensation. In the course of this workshop the survivors worked toward separating these paired associations and, in doing so, freed their bodies and increased their abilities to recognize and respond to healthy sexuality.

The next session focused on how sexuality can be addressed through the use of a survivor's dreams and creative imagery. Rita, who had been molested in childhood by a neighbor, suffered in her marriage from inhibited sexual desire. In this particular session, she described a dream of a barren desert, scrubby and apparently lifeless. In the distance, a cactus flower was pushing up toward the light, against the restraints of the rough soil. Rita said that her body felt as desolate as this barren land. The flower seemed to express a desire for intimacy with her husband. Rita danced as a struggling flower trying to break out and reach toward the sky. Her conflicts were expressed by her own image of the impacted soil. With Rita's permission to touch her, I placed my palms on her upper back and took on the role of the soil pushing down as Rita struggled upward. When her ambivalence about her own freedom was externalized, Rita broke free to devote her full attention to a dance of positive desire.

In the sessions that followed, Rita focused on the results of having numbed her body and cut off her feelings. She was encouraged to dance images that helped her struggling flower grow. Images from nature of sensuality, receptivity, and fluidity helped her to liberate locked up sexuality. Over time, she was able to bring her newly developing freedoms into the intimacy of her marriage.

Conclusions

Success in helping the survivor use her body as a therapy tool depends on the dance therapist's commitment to the curative power of movement. For many survivors, "letting go to dance" has become inexorably linked with the terror of loss of control experienced during the abuse. This association can paralyze movement in spite of the survivors' will. The survivor relies on the therapist to help her resist her pull away from her body. She also learns from the dance therapist that her power and control do not depend on withholding movement; rather, her power is in which parts of her body she chooses to move and how she moves them.

When a survivor participates in the dance therapy process, hope and positive feelings about her body can be restored. She is able to bridge her thoughts and feelings with action and to reclaim her body as her own. She becomes more expressive, more creative, and physically stronger in her own eyes as she develops feelings of control and power. From an improved relationship to her body she finds her way to create a more healthful and satisfying life.

3

Mobilizing Battered Women:
A Creative Step Forward

Meg Chang and Fern Leventhal

The battered woman has received a great deal of attention in recent years. Domestic violence, however, continues to be widespread and is devastating to all involved.[1] A "battered woman is a woman who is repeatedly subjected to any forceful physical or psychological behavior by a man in order to coerce her to do something he wants her to do without any concern for her rights" (Walker, 1979, p. xv).[2] Victims of domestic violence must be able to take action if they are to remedy learned patterns of helplessness, ambivalence, and inactivity. Dance and creative movement offer a paradigm for action that can help women in danger take the steps necessary to reorganize their lives.

Physical violence, emotional abuse, financial deprivation, and sexual coercion all constitute battering. Although different forms may occur separately or in combination, physical abuse is the most obvious—as evidenced by black eyes, bruises, and broken bones. However, less visible physical manifestations include kicking, slapping, choking, shoving, and destruction of the battered person's property. Emotional abuse may include suggestions of physical violence such as threats to kill, maim, or disable. Even subtle forms of intimidation and humiliation serve to undermine the woman's self-confidence and independence. Threats against other family members are also common and are intended to induce fear and compliance. Financial abuse, which is characterized by both domination and deprivation, occurs at all socioeconomic levels. Enforced by the threat of violence, this abuse effectively reinforces a woman's dependency. Economic abuse can take several forms. A battered woman may be forced to be the sole financial support for the family. Or, conversely, she may be prevented from earning, or having, any money of her own, or from having any financial responsibility or knowledge. Finally, sexual abuse includes violent and coercive sex aimed at proving domination. Other more subtle forms of sexual abuse include humiliation, seduction, and manipulation.

Unable to alter the man's behavior and burdened by the effects of constant abuse, the battered woman perceives few alternatives for changing her life. She becomes increasingly passive and compliant as she is repeatedly subjected to situations in which she cannot predict or control the violence. In time she internalizes the role of victim and accepts the inevitability of the abusive relationship. Thus, "the process of victimization is perpetuated to the point of psychological paralysis" (Walker, 1979, p. 43).

Pervasive apprehension and paralyzing terror become a battered woman's chronic response to threats of abuse and violence. During an attack the woman's physical sensation becomes blunted; she develops the ability to cut off all feeling (Walker, 1979). Because she is unable to control the violence or defend herself, she psycho-physically detaches or dissociates herself from the experience.

Dissociation allows the woman to isolate herself from her fear, rage, and hopelessness. At times, she may only be conscious of her feelings of love for the abuser. Her intensely negative feelings may split off from her consciousness and be denied (Paley, 1988). This splitting of her awareness inhibits the battered woman's ability to respond appropriately to signs of danger. Moreover, uncomfortable emotions such as anger, sadness, and loss may be projected onto the abuser (Gillman, 1980). By assigning her feelings to the abuser, she minimizes her experience and thereby the ability to protect herself. Dissociation and projection reinforce the tendency toward denial and the magical belief that the abuse won't happen again. It is this type of thinking that becomes a stumbling block in treatment.

Over time, a battered woman accepts the abuser's view of "reality," seeing herself as he describes her—worthless, stupid, ugly, or undesirable. As her self-esteem is undermined, the ability to make autonomous decisions declines and she begins to accept her partner as all-powerful and all-knowing. A woman involved with an abusive partner wants to believe that he is deeply sorry, that he will change, and that the "honeymoon" period following the abuse will prevail (Walker, 1979).

Ambivalence, a prevalent factor in the psychology of battered women, is expressed as indecision about whether to stay or to leave the relationship (Rounsaville, Lipton, & Bieber, 1979). This ambivalence is fueled partially by feelings of helplessness, lack of a strong self-identity, and fear of change. In addition, lack of financial independence is a practical consideration that reinforces the difficulties of leaving (NiCarthy, 1982). Lowered self-esteem and embarrassment may prevent a woman from seeking assistance from friends, relatives, or professionals. Ashamed by physical injuries and reluctant to discuss her situation, the woman retreats. Further isolation may be induced by the abuser's pathological jealousy, which serves to quarantine the woman from even casual contacts (Walker, 1979). Friends and family, often frightened by the violence and reluctant to become caught up in the victim's ambivalence, withdraw their support. Social seclusion further tips the balance of power toward the oppressor.

The cycle of violence increases the woman's belief that she has no control over the events in her life. Her dependence and loss of control may be reinforced by social institutions—law-enforcement authorities, the legal system, or welfare agencies—which may be either ineffective or unresponsive to her needs (Schecter, 1987).

Dance/Movement Therapy

Decreasing Isolation

The ability to embody independent actions and experience the conscious choice to move is a matter of vital importance to victims of abuse. Creative movement combined with therapy motivates victims to act; it addresses patterns of isolation, helplessness, ambivalence, and immobilization. Breaking a battered woman's isolation is a primary consideration. It is crucial that a woman's first contact in therapy reinforce the fact that she is not alone in her distress. Often disconnected from friends and family, women benefit from hearing the experiences of others. Indeed, "the realization that their situation is not uncommon reduces their shame and feelings of personal inadequacy" (Lewis, 1983, p. 56).

A creative and expressive group process that unites women around a common theme can reduce self-blame and decrease alienation. For example, in one group, which was co-led with a playwright,[3] the women enacted the Harriet Tubman story. Tubman escaped both slavery and an abusive husband, and became one of the legendary conductors of the underground railroad. Inspired by her heroic story, the women dramatically integrated aspects of Tubman's tale with their own tragic stories. The dances that resulted traced their long and arduous journeys from slavery to freedom.

Confronting Day-to-Day Problems

Expression and catharsis alone are not enough to repair the lives of battered women and their families. Faced with catastrophic life situations, practical solutions to daily problems may prove elusive. Identification of these day-to-day problems, and their solutions, often emerge from the creative process, however. For example, when the therapist suggested to the group an image of "reaching for what you want," one woman fantasized about escaping from her abusive boyfriend. She had often spoken to the group about wanting to end the relationship but she had been unable to. During her dance she reached toward an open window and moved her arms as if she wanted "wings to fly away." But her arms tired quickly and she remained fixed to the floor—suddenly aware of the impossibility of her wish. The therapist took this opportunity to help the woman confront her fantasies of escape. She was asked to consider more realistic options for distancing herself from her boyfriend's destructive behavior. After some discussion, the client realized that she could begin to remove herself from her boyfriend by altering her work schedule and, in this way, gather her strength and plan the next move.

As illustrated above, the therapist can help the client confront her unrealistic psycho-physical distortions as they emerge in the dance and movement process. Knowledge gained through the observation of movement patterns can be reflected back to the mover in an empathic and constructive way. Moreover, the mover herself will discover insights in response to her physical sensations and expressions (Leventhal & Chang, 1991). Although underlying psychological damage may take years to be recognized and resolved, immediate and protective measures safeguard a woman's life and well-being.

Broadening Movement and Life Choices

Broadening movement patterns is another way of introducing new behaviors. Movement increases the battered woman's range of action and interaction. Living in a constrained relationship can lead to rigid movement patterns as well as limited coping styles. It follows that expanding the individual's movement repertoire is directly linked to changes in self-concept and interpersonal dynamics (North, 1972). For example, in a session a battered woman may be surprised by her own strength when she is encouraged by the therapist to push against a partner. Finding her strength, she begins to accept the therapist's observation that she is not the "pushover" she thought herself to be. This affirmation enables her to interact more assertively with the important figures in her life and begin to perceive herself more positively. Similarly, a woman who feels weak and helpless can mobilize feelings of personal power and a desire to fight back when provided with simple everyday props, such as small hand weights or a tennis racket. When props are used during improvisational dance, they tend to increase muscle activity and thereby expand the person's total commitment to her actions (F. Levy, Personal Communication: Oct. 12th, 1994). Bartky (1980) states that "without the active use of weight, there is little hope that these women will ever be able to stand up for themselves" (p. 135).

Exploring the use of space can also bring about a change in both behavior and self-perception. Schmais (1974) states that, "changes often occur in movement before they occur in other areas" (p. 11). This is exemplified in one client's discovery of a link between her movement patterns and her life choices. The woman said that she enjoyed the improvisational movement sessions because they were "freeing" and seemed to help her deal with her restricted posture and physical tension. In one session, during an improvisation, she raised her arms in full extension, exploring the space above her, as if for the first time. She said, "I'm stretching towards a new life." Then she spoke of her many interests that had not been realized during her marriage and made plans to contact important people from her past. This woman's small, yet realistic, change should not be minimized. It is through these manageable steps that a battered women can raise her self-esteem and reduce feelings of helplessness.

The technique of mirroring an individual's movement can be used to establish trust and promote a therapeutic alliance. It may be contraindicated as a long-term intervention, however, as it can reinforce dependency on the leader. Like all individuals in treatment, battered women move through stages of growth. As their needs change and mature, the treatment approach must shift to meet the new demands (Huston, 1984). The importance of the battered woman's increased independence and autonomous functioning must be recognized and validated. "Victims of violence need to be encouraged to take control of their lives, and learning to share control of their therapy is a beginning step toward that goal" (Walker, 1989, p. 701). Though the therapist has a responsibility to provide the tools and information the client needs to change her situation, insistence on any course of action can reinforce passivity. A battered woman must be encouraged to generate her own options, assess alternatives, and seek her own solutions (Bowen, 1982).

Clients who have become conditioned to rigid and hierarchical modes of relating may react to movement directives with either compliance or rebellion. Incorporating an approach that encourages self-directed action not only defuses the issues surrounding control but also taps sources of individual choice and creativity. Exercises that explore emotionally charged, contrasting movements such as "near and far," "up and down," "push and pull" stimulate the expression of individual concerns and conflicts. While moving, a battered woman discovers her own images, metaphors, and associations. She is helped to make meaningful connections between the contrasting movements and emotions explored in her dance and similar situations in her life. For example, a woman's push/pull movement can become a way to explore her ambivalent feelings toward her abuser. As the client responds, without superimposed movement from the therapist or group, she contacts her own unique sources of initiation and generates a personal "route to change" (Blanche Evan, Personal Communication, October 1982).

Choosing Movement Directives

Thoughtfully articulated movement directives are essential, as illustrated in the following vignette. After the warm-up, the therapist noticed that several women were kicking. In an attempt to reflect the group's feelings, the therapist suggested that the women "kick *him* away." The reaction of the group to this interpretation was to perform a few explosive movements that quickly diminished into unfocused, peripheral actions. The intensity of feeling that seemed to be developing prior to the movement directive dissipated and the movements came to a premature and unsatisfying closure. The therapist, after reflecting on what had happened to the group, came to the conclusion that her suggestion to "kick him away" overdefined and overdirected the action of the women. When the kicking resurfaced, the therapist supported the group's physical intentions by saying, "make noise with your feet and legs and use all the space in the room." This simple movement directive resulted in an exuberant dance. A group rhythm eventually spread as the women joined in each other's expressions of strength. The less interpretive suggestion emphasized expanding the women's ability to express themselves fully without burdening their movements with an analysis or preconceived formulation. Premature interpretation of the client's nonverbal experience "is liable to foreclose individual process" (Mackay, 1989, p. 300) and rob abused women of the opportunity to make meaning out of their own symbolic expression. The women must be encouraged to stay with their feelings long enough to identify and own them for themselves.

Patterns of self-denigration, rumination, and rigid thinking dominate the battered woman's thought processes. For these women "taking a step forward" is much more than a figure of speech. Accustomed to passivity and immobilization, taking a step in any direction can be frustratingly difficult and even unimaginable. As a battered woman is helped to experiment with a variation of "steps," she begins to see herself as capable of action and change.

The creativity and activity inherent in dance can counteract ingrained patterns of compliance and immobilization. One woman, in a short-term group, described how she responded when arguing with her lover. "Something happens to me when he starts yelling at me. I know I should just get up and leave, but my feet are frozen." With encouragement from the therapist she was able to express in movement the feeling of immobility. When the woman experienced the physical sensation of being unable to move, changes in her breath and muscle tone became apparent. After exploring the sensation of paralyzed legs and the thoughts and associations that arose in response to this sensation, she was then asked how she might move her legs if they weren't frozen. Such directives are most effective when derived from the client's own body actions and physical metaphors. Creative dance, improvisation, and role-playing of powerful feelings all facilitate safe expression of effect. Levy (1992) describes creative and expressive dance as coming under the domain of the ego and, as such, something that "can help individuals to experience and express repressed traumas and other forbidden and frightening thoughts and feelings" (p. 37) in a constructive manner.

Building Emotional Tolerence

Even when the immediate danger to the battered woman has been reduced, tendencies toward dissociation continue to distance her from overwhelming feelings of fear and rage. In the course of the abuse, a basic level of trust in herself, in intimate relationships, and in the environment has been lost. An abused woman can, however, be helped to reinhabit her body through gradually building tolerance to the physical and emotional sensations that she previously disowned. For example, practicing conscious awareness of breath is most often a nonthreatening intervention that is both physically and psychologically stabilizing. Psycho-physical awareness can help a woman monitor, and possibly manage, her anxiety. If, during dance/movement, an abused woman suddenly becomes conscious of her previously split-off feelings, panic may ensue. Focusing on her breath and immediate body sensations is a way to return to the present while allowing fears from the past to be investigated.

In the following example, however, a leader's suggestion to try a simple relaxation and breathing exercise had an unexpected outcome. A group of battered women, not currently in life-threatening situations, were complaining of anxiety and insomnia. The leader asked them to close their eyes and begin to breathe deeply. Within minutes, one woman said that she felt panicked. Another woman described her phobias of riding the subway; a third revealed that on many days she felt unable to leave her apartment. Because of the group's difficulty in maintaining internal controls, the leader told the group to focus on their surroundings. She suggested that they notice the presence of others, pay attention to the temperature of the air against their skin, and feel the chair under them. This was an attempt to bring the women into the present where they were safe. In the discussion that ensued, they openly shared their own private strategies for managing their intense and persistent fears.

It is important to help the abused women experience a continuum of physical and emotional sensation. The therapist, however, needs to be aware that relaxation exercises and cathartic movement, designed to put individuals in touch with their emotions and bodily sensations, may, in fact, restimulate terrifying feelings and force the abused woman to retreat again into denial or dissociation. Moreover, as the client gets in touch with her fury, including her own feelings of violence toward her perpetrator, she may become so alarmed by her own aggression that she leaves treatment. Toward the other extreme, movements that express letting go or giving in (indulgent sensations) may evoke feelings of engulfment, loss of autonomy, helplessness, and shame. "When the work is deep, each experiential phase may uncover another layer of experience or aspect of self, often for the first time in a recognizable form. Time should be allowed between phases for quiet and natural integration of what has gone on before" (Mackay, 1989, p. 300). It is, therefore, important that the client determine the pacing and intensity of the nonverbal experience. By gradually expressing her feelings, the battered woman gains control of her internal processes and senses her own power.

Movement Feedback

Presenting the women with information about their movement patterns can enhance their understanding of themselves. For example, with feedback from the therapist, one woman realized how she continued to act out her ambivalence toward her own independence. The woman said she felt as though she was "running in circles." As she spoke, she frantically twirled her hands in the air while her torso and legs remained immobilized. Her hand twirling occurred as she elaborated on a costly legal situation with her ex-lover, a situation that was perpetuating the psychological abuse characteristic of their 20-year relationship. The client became aware of her ambivalent feelings when the contradiction between her gestures and posture was brought to her attention. She realized that by participating as a passive victim in the legal struggle, she was maintaining the abusive relationship.

Countertransference

When treating abused women the therapist needs to recognize the influence of her own preconceptions, associations, and fantasies. The therapist's feelings about the patient, her countertransference, can be a "trap" that diminishes the effectiveness of treatment and contributes to therapist burn-out (Chu, 1988). Identification with the "victim" can lead to a blurring of the boundaries between client and therapist. Therapists with rescue fantasies may direct clients toward premature decisions. If the therapist gets caught up in a power struggle with the patient, reenactment of the abusive relationship may occur. This may stimulate hostility or dependency from the patient. In addition, avoidance of the battered woman's anger and rage, due to the therapist's discomfort with these emotions, can immobilize both therapist and client, as illustrated in the following vignette.

Jane bitterly recounted her history of abuse. Her hostile diatribe was accompanied by shortness of breath, muscular rigidity, and strong, intense jabs with her hands. "How can I get rid of my anger at my ex-husband? He ruined my life, running up thousands of dollars of debt...I had cancer when I was pregnant...I feel like my life is a deck of cards that could fall apart if any one part is touched." Jane's story was an especially dramatic one. The therapist's impulse was to rescue her and resolve her problems quickly. In an attempt to help Jane "get rid of" her anger, the leader suggested that the walking warm-up "begin with a little kick."

In response to this directive, Jane grew uncomfortable, increasingly tense, and was unable to move. She angrily demanded that the therapist help her to bend her locked knees. The therapist, intimidated by Jane's rage, was surprised to find herself immobilized. Like the client, the therapist suddenly felt unable to move her legs. Shifting her attention to movement cues from another, more responsive, group member the therapist gave the directive, "use your whole foot when you walk." Jane responded by retracting her toes, locking her jaw, and eventually withdrawing from the group. Under attack, the therapist felt blocked and was not able to assist Jane with appropriate movement interventions. The therapist's inability to quickly monitor her own feelings prevented her from helping the client to feel safe and accepted.

Because of the intensity of the emotions and stories that battered women bring to treatment, countertransference is frequently, often suddenly, evoked. In addition, when the abused woman is unable to recognize her own feelings, she may project them onto the therapist. Analyzing this phenomenon provides clues to treatment and thus becomes an extremely important tool in the therapist–client relationship.

Conclusions

"Abused women may be able to accept superficially that they are people of worth, but it takes positive experiences over time for them to internalize this concept" (Ibrahim & Herr, 1987 p. 247). With repeated validation, the battered woman can internalize a sense of herself as someone capable of action, achievement, and love. Therapeutic change can be assessed by alterations in mobility, perceptions, patterns of behavior, and interaction. The ultimate effectiveness of treatment is measured by the choices a woman makes in her life.

Only the woman herself can judge what is best for her. Whether she leaves the abusive situation or remains, treatment gives her the ego strength and emotional support to mitigate the abuse and increase her safety. The physical and action-oriented approach of dance/movement therapy promotes a battered woman's pschodynamic growth while supplying a much needed dynamic—*the ability to move!*

4

"I Can't Have Me if I Don't Have You": Working with the Borderline Personality

Joan Lavender and Wendy Sobelman

This chapter presents an approach to the treatment of patients with borderline personality disorder. Historically, the term "borderline" (Knight & Freidman, 1954) referred to a mental status that fluctuated between neurotic problems and severe mental states in which there was a temporary loss of the ability to perceive reality. Due largely to the contributions of numerous psychodynamic thinkers, including Kernberg (1975), Adler and Buie (1973), Giovacchini (1982), and Masterson (1972), the classification of borderline personality has developed into a diagnosis in its own right.

Diagnosis

DSM-IV: Behavioral Manifestations

Borderline personality disorder is characterized by a pattern of instability of mood, interpersonal relationships, and self-image. These patterns usually begin in early adulthood and are pervasive. Features of the diagnosis include unstable intense interpersonal relationships characterized by overidealization and devaluation, impulsivity, and self-destructive behaviors such as overeating, shoplifting, substance abuse, and self-mutilation. Affective instability, lack of control of anger, recurrent suicidal threats, identity disturbances, chronic feelings of emptiness and frantic efforts to avoid abandonment all may be present (American Psychiatric Association, 1994).

The borderline individual often lives life as a helpless victim on a roller coaster ride, anticipating the next crisis while barely surviving previous ones. For example, when Margie was discharged from a psychiatric hospitalization, she ended a quarrel with her parents by cutting her wrist with a razor. She was rehospitalized and immediately after the next discharge she got intoxicated and "found herself" in bed with a stranger. She reported that she had hoped for affection and was shocked to be expected to have sex. After this incident Margie was evicted from her apartment and began a cycle of anorexia that developed into a full-blown medical crisis, which again precipitated hospitalization. At this point she had to anticipate her therapist's vacation. Her anxiety increased and she put her fist through a brick wall, displaying the bloody knuckles to her therapist before he left on vacation.

Kernberg (1975) establishes the borderline personality within populations he defines as having a "lower level character pathology." This determination is made on the basis of three areas: poor tolerance for emotional states, poor impulse control, and an underdeveloped ability to sublimate. Sublimation is understood as the capacity to deal with frustration by the use of constructive or symbolic activities. Together these deficits may give borderline individuals a childish quality. The behavior of adult patients is often reminiscent of the stages and crises of early childhood.

The following is an example of all three deficits as they emerged in an initial stage of treatment. In a group session a patient was unable to sustain her attention long enough to complete a brief structured movement exercise. The therapist suggested she choose a satisfying way of moving her arms, then develop the movement, and bring it to a close. The patient began in a perfunctory manner, but the act of moving itself seemed to fan her emotions. Within a few moments her movements became erotic. When she became aware of sexual sensations, she could neither verbalize her discomfort, nor modulate the intensity or quality of the movement. Seemingly unable to contain the sensations the movement generated, she felt she had no option but to flee the room.

Although this individual never lost a basic sense of reality, as might a schizophrenic patient in such a situation, her momentary loss of control made the exercise impossible. It would be typical for a borderline patient to feel humiliated after this "failure" at a task that, on its surface, seemed simple and straightforward.

Borderline patients suffer from a chronic instability that characterizes every aspect of their lives. They lack a single, cohesive sense of identity needed to make life predictable. A healthy individual has a sense of continuity of self.

This continuity, or what is generally meant by the terms character or personality, enables individuals to adapt to changes in life situations. Identity confusion, a feeling of uncertainty regarding the reliability of one's identity, causes the borderline patient to feel and behave in unpredictable ways.

The Abandonment Crisis

Since the term borderline was first offered (Knight, 1953), theories of human development have attempted to explain the genesis of the phenomenon. Mahler, Pine, and Bergman's (1975) research, based on movement observations of infants and young children and their mothers, can be used as a developmental model to understand the origins of behavior. The researchers describe a series of hallmarks that emerge around the 18th month of life. At this time the toddler confronts a dilemma, the resolution of which (or lack thereof) may determine a lifelong problem. This dilemma is termed "rapprochement crisis." It refers to a psychological predicament in which the toddler is faced with integrating two radically different internal attitudes toward her own sense of identity. The conflict manifests in behavior that is alternately demanding and rejecting—the "terrible twos."

The child's first sense of identity is of herself as expansive and capable, newly able to move around without the physical support of a caretaker. This necessarily grandiose little person uses her growing set of emotional and cognitive skills in the service of making the world bend to her wishes. The sense of omnipotence is an illusion, however, as the child's emotional buoyancy and physical daring is, of course, dependent on the support of a caretaker whose responsibility, ideally, is not to puncture the illusion.

An opposite mental state occurs when the child needs to return to her caretaker for physical support, emotional affirmation, or to share in a state of joy. Such refueling is essential if the toddler is to maintain a feeling of competence. If the child is unable to accomplish this task, either by some lack on the part of the caretaker, some physical handicap in the child, or an external circumstance, she may experience the loss of the illusion. Grandiosity and vitality are then replaced by a depleted sense of self and a fear of exploration. Alternations of rage and clinging behavior may also appear. This dilemma is called an "abandonment crisis" (Mahler, Pine, & Bergman, 1975). Although normal and expectable, it must be handled with sensitivity.

The adult borderline patient, like the 2-year-old, presents a range of behavior that fluctuates rapidly between regressive disintegration and nearly adequate behavior. Such clients face alternating fears of abandonment and engulfment. These rapprochement issues may be enacted by individuals as well as by groups. On the one hand, circle dances that emphasize the loss of self in a communal experience, however brief, can raise fears of loss of autonomy. On the other hand, dances that heighten a sense of individuality can evoke fears of aloneness and isolation. The perpetual shifts, from autonomy to refueling, require ongoing attention by the therapist as exemplified by the process described below.

A group of patients, who had developed a sense of cohesion, asked the therapist if they could move to a larger room, a gym. The therapist consented. In the gym the patients devised their own dance structures and brought in their own music. They ran and leapt through the space. Suddenly one day, a member asked that the group return to the old circle formation and take turns leading. Another patient said incredulously, "But it's how we began in this group, when we did that all the time!"

The patient's protest went no further, as the other members agreed to revert to the familiar circle formation. Eventually they even asked to return to the smaller room. Initially, the therapist was disappointed; she was aware of feeling she had "set them free." They had moved away from her and had expressed a sense of joyful autonomy. The therapist then realized that she had overlooked the fears and vulnerabilities inherent in independent action for this population. The patients were indeed expressing a need to refuel.

Borderline Defenses

The identification of specific defenses (LaPlanche & Pontalis, 1973) is another perspective from which to clarify the phenomenon of borderline personality. A defense is an unconscious mechanism used to protect the individual from perceived danger or discomfort (Moore & Fine, 1968). Kernberg (1975) refers to the use of four defenses—splitting, primitive idealization, denial, and projective identification—as the hallmarks of this disorder.

Splitting is based on a normal developmental phenomenon in which experiences that feel good or satisfying are segregated from those that feel distinctly bad or frustrating. These split experiences can affect the infant's sense of self so that she develops an image of herself when frustrated as "bad" and when satisfied as "good." These impressions of self are termed self-representations (LaPlanche & Pontalis, 1973). The two segregated states eventually become integrated, so that a person experiences herself, as well as the external world, as neither entirely good nor entirely bad, but as a mixture of both. Kernberg (1975) believes that the borderline individual may be born with excessive aggression, which may further trigger a split in self-perception. This excess diminishes the child's capacity to integrate satisfying and depriving experiences, as well as good and bad images of herself. As a result, the child's ego is poorly developed, and a unified sense of identity is not achieved.

A patient entered a therapy session full of ambition to start her career as a professional dancer. She could barely contain her pleasure in learning structured exercises, and was shocked when other members of the group were reluctant to improvise. Her aggressive enthusiasm had the effect of alienating others. In the next session, she invented an excuse for being unable to move at all. She persuaded the therapist to let her sit in the corner of the room where she made snide comments about how this form of therapy was a waste of time. This patient could not combine her two attitudes toward the treatment, nor could she comprehend how her own attitude shifted. It eventually became clear that the patient was excessively sensitive to slight nonverbal signs from the therapist, signs she interpreted as encouraging or discouraging her involvement and ambition. She distorted the meaning of the therapist's movements and took them as signs of her potential success or failure in the session. In other words, she was not able to maintain an integrated sense of self—good and bad—without clear confirmation by the therapist.

Denial refers to the unconscious rejection of an aspect of reality. A borderline patient may deny the emotional relevance of something she has experienced, while maintaining an accurate perception of the facts of reality. Denial should not be mistaken for lying, which is also common in this population.

Primitive idealization refers to the child's fantasy of an all-powerful parent, a fantasy that gives the child the belief that she can be protected from a dangerous world (Kernberg, 1975). The borderline adult, who uses primitive idealization as a defense, may be attempting to preserve a good feeling toward another.

Projection occurs when qualities, feeling, or wishes that the person rejects as a part of herself are attributed to others. In *projective identification* (LaPlanche & Pontalis, 1973), the individual takes a disturbing aspect of her own personality and projects it to the other person. However, unable to successfully leave these qualities behind, she finds herself compelled to control them in the other person. While projection is considered a common defense mechanism, projective identification is considered a hallmark of borderline phenomena.

Clinicians often report the uncanny sense of being "caught up" in a patient's process of projective identification. A therapist who is the object of such an identification frequently feels that some unpleasant aspect of her own personality has become exaggerated and is the target of a patient's relentless criticism. Such criticism may eventually cause the therapist to feel exposed, overwhelmed, and retaliatory, as exemplified in the vignette below.

A female patient suffered from extreme insecurity and awkwardness about movement. Her defense was to behave in a divisive and critical manner toward the therapist and fellow patients. During one session she compared the group's dance to her memory of normal children laughing at retarded children playing in a schoolyard. This comment had an unconscious impact on the therapist who, over time, found herself feeling uncharacteristically awkward and unable to improvise. The therapist's resistance to movement became so intense that entire sessions were spent talking rather than moving. The discussions had an avoidant quality, as the therapist noticed her own reluctance to design movement structures for the group. The feeling of paralysis was pervasive. The therapist noticed that she was experiencing a deep sense of incompetence.

One day, when this particular patient was absent, the therapist found herself countering the group's paralysis with humorous suggestions about ways to start moving. Because the group members feared looking "stupid, silly, dumb, or too sexy," the therapist began an awkward and silly dance, inviting them to join her with the words, "Let's get it over with!" It was discovered that certain members of the group were natural comics and mimes. The dances became hilarious. The group moved together as each dancer initiated her own and also copied others' outrageous movements. The humor released the fear, even for the most inhibited members of the group.

The phenomenon of projective identification took months to analyze. Only when other staff identified a similar experience with the absence of the same patient did the therapist begin to realize that she was involved in such a process. Through her analysis of this phenomenon she was able to appreciate the extent of her patient's contempt for herself and how it had been projected onto the therapist. At this point, the therapist felt free to function in her role again.

Following this insight, and through the group process, members were able to tell the patient the effect that her attitude had had on them. In addition, the patient was helped to make a meaningful connection between her behavior in the group and the contemptuous and tyrannizing effect she had had on her own family. She stated, " I wasn't going to let them move ahead if I was so stuck."

The mechanism of projective identification may temporarily result in a loss of self-esteem and confidence in the therapist's professional identity. Supervision often helps to regain perspective and at times may be essential when treating a borderline patient.

Kohut's Selfobject Transference

Borderline individuals have serious difficulty with emotional and behavioral regulation. It follows that such persons may seek others to function as regulators for them. The use of relationships with others to provide such regulation is what Kohut (1977) means by a "selfobject" function. The spelling of "selfobject" is intended to indicate that the other person is perceived not in his or her own right, but essentially as an object for, or psychological extension of, the self. The individual who is cast by the borderline in the selfobject role supplies regulation of emotions and self-esteem, as well as an overall sense of aliveness and cohesion. The borderline who continues to require selfobject relations is unable to modulate her own needs. She often becomes possessive and makes excessive demands toward the significant other on whom she feels dependent. The borderline patient engaged in such an emotional relationship will idealize the significant other (selfobject) when she feels her needs are being met. The idealization, however, abruptly shifts to devaluation, aloofness, contempt, or rage if the individual is disappointed and disillusioned with the object. The borderline person needs constant admiration from the selfobject; criticism evokes an icy grandiose response or intensified somatic concerns (Kohut, 1971).

The following is an example of what happens when the therapist, previously idealized, becomes the recipient of the patient's intense envy and hate. A 68-year-old female patient extended her arms as she danced toward the therapist. In the past the patient had demanded much individual time with the therapist. She used this time to describe how she was mistreated by others. The patient often made complimentary statements about the therapist's appearance and youth, but also resented the therapist for not having spent enough time exclusively with her. In her dance, as her bright crimson fingernails came dangerously close to the therapist's face, the patient smiled and said, "Those green eyes...I could scratch them out!" In this moment, the patient's insatiable needs combined with her excessive aggression to form intense feelings of envy.

Selfobject relationships often involve coercive demands that the object conform to the needs of the patient. In extreme cases, the selfobject may be held responsible for the life of the patient, as in threats of suicide. Such behavior can be viewed as a form of manipulation to gain control of the object. Patients with such intense needs to control others are frequently unable to be alone. When alone, they feel a devastating sense of emptiness that can easily move them to compulsive and addictive behaviors.

The need for a selfobject relationship may be especially important in the treatment of patients with sexual and physical abuse histories. In fact, it has been substantiated that the majority of patients with the diagnosis of borderline personality disorder have such a history (Herman, 1992). This has interfered with their ability to trust others. Self-loathing impairs their capacity to care for themselves. These patients often resort to self-harming behaviors including suicidality, self-mutilation and eating disorders in order to regulate intolerable feeling states. The establishment of a selfobject transference in the therapeutic relationship can help to provide the holding and self-soothing elements lacking in the individual, as illustrated in the following vignette.

Mackenzie was referred to the day center following a serious suicide attempt precipitated by an experience of abandonment and her growing awareness that she had been a victim of incest. Her presentation was remarkable in the following way: she did not appear depressed but was completely out of touch with herself, she was depersonalized most of the time. To cope with the discomfort of depersonalization and dissociation, she abused herself through cutting and burning her skin. Strangely enough, this behavior provided her with some temporary relief.

Mackenzie's relationship with the dance therapist was dependent and idealizing. The therapist, in turn, was aware of her own strong protective and maternal feelings toward Mackenzie. She found herself articulating reactions of alarm and concern over her destructive behavior. Mackenzie's attitude toward her own dangerous acts and lack of self-care was one of indifference. It was as if she could not be bothered to protect herself or even to care where she would eat, sleep, or live.

Mackenzie's main problem in relationships was her inability to maintain her autonomy. She would force others to care for her. Without this caring, she would become isolated and depersonalized. During the course of treatment, this pattern of intense need for another—a selfobject relationship—was brought to the therapist. During this process Mackenzie created a personal symbol of a "defective kitten left to die." Over a period of many months she dealt with her disgust around her own neediness and sense of being damaged by creating dances around this symbol. The dances alternated between expressions of revulsion and compassion for the hurt kitten.

The therapist utilized the power of the selfobject transference and Mackenzie's creativity to endorse her compassion, not only for the kitten but also for herself, and legitimize her early, unmet needs. Through creative improvisation, which was always encouraged, and discussion, Mackenzie's feelings of need became less humiliating and more acceptable.

Separations from the therapist were at first very hard for Mackenzie but became more tolerable when she was able to internalize the therapist's self-soothing functions. Instead of her characteristic cutting and self-abuse, she began to use dance to soothe herself even when alone. When treatment ended, she was able to acknowledge that she could take over her own self-care and that suicide was no longer an option.

It is important to note that borderline patients, after experiencing dance improvisation in the groups, often begin to dance at home. This appears to help regulate the intensity of their emotions and to replace the need to physically abuse themselves.

Movement Syndromes and the Creative Process

The phenomenon of play emerges naturally in human beings when a minimal standard of secure attachment to a caretaker has been established. Healthy play in young children allows them to move freely from imagination to reality within a protective environment. Bowlby (1969) described a disturbance in the play of children that he called "pathology of play." Terr (1990), in a similar vein, differentiated between normal play and the play of children who have undergone traumatic experiences; she describes the qualities of the latter as grim, monotonous, and with little variation.

Likewise, individuals with borderline traits do not have an inner sense of security, hence their capacity to become invested in playful or creative endeavors is limited. Improvisational dance is a kind of play. The dancer must allow herself access to the elements of her inner life—imagination, thoughts, sensory experience, memory, and so on, as she expresses herself through the physical abilities and limitations of her body. Such movement explorations are intrinsically satisfying when the dancer can express some aspect of her inner life in external forms.

The authors have noted three movement syndromes that obstruct the dancer in her attempt to produce satisfying improvisations. The pressure to discharge feelings directly through action, before they are successfully symbolized, is one movement syndrome. (See example of patient who ran out of the room.) Another syndrome is dance that is monotonous, compulsively repetitive, or constricted. Some patients insist on repeating ballet steps in a perfunctory fashion. Stereotyped movement defends the dancer from the danger of succumbing to a chaotic inner life, but also prevents him/her from working through conflicts. Finally, some patients produce dances that are wish fulfillment's—highly stylized and emotionally detached attempts to portray naive and romanticized human relationships. These dances may be thought of as flight from the difficulties and complexity of reality. Such improvisations frequently involve the dancer in fantasies of extraordinary abilities or of specialness of some sort. It is the authors' impression that patients who prefer this type of dance frequently have difficulty accepting the fact that it takes hard work to achieve one's goals in life.

For example, one male patient was only interested in dancing when the opportunity to be carried on the shoulders of other patients was presented. He was unwilling to do the hard work of lifting others or, for that matter, of developing his own muscles to the point where he could use his own strength. He was reluctant to discuss the situation in the group. Eventually, he revealed a childhood wish retained into adulthood of being carried around like a king. He offered this memory with shy embarrassment. The patient was then able to discuss how his lifelong wish to be treated like a king had adversely affected his ability to work cooperatively with others.

Somatic Concerns

Borderline patients are often preoccupied with somatic complaints and concerns that are hypochondriacal in nature. In addition, these patients may harbor misinformation about how the body actually works, looks, and feels. Their complaints frequently reveal distortions of the body image and these distortions can hamper their ability to move (Schilder, 1950). For example, an anorexic patient believed that there were "hills" inside her thighs that made her appear misshapen; the hills were actually an image she developed in response to touching the area of her thighs that contained the most sensitive bundles of musculature and nerve endings. When the therapist offered her an explanation, the patient became more relaxed about her own body and her movements.

Another patient, with a history of physical abuse, had difficulty initiating movement from any part of her body other than hands or feet. When asked by the therapist to create "movement that starts from the center of your body," she became upset and said she could sense only a "gaping hole" in the center of her body. Numbness is a somatic form of denial. This individual, in order not to feel the pain of her abuse, had blocked out all sensations in the center of her torso.

When a history of sexual abuse is present, an intense negative attitude directed toward the particular body parts that were abused is common. One woman, who bound her breasts because she felt they were too large, described a history of sexual abuse. Her precocious physical development was used as an excuse by her perpetrator to justify his behavior. This patient was left feeling that her feminine features were responsible for her abuse.

Another patient believed that he looked like an 8-year-old boy when in fact he was muscularly well-developed and six feet tall. He was aware that his body image was distorted, but the distortion was persistent and pervasive. In summary, the somatic concerns of the borderline patient are substantial and can be addressed directly through the modality of movement.

Treatment

Goals and Techniques of Treatment

As with all patients it is important for the therapist to be explicit and descriptive regarding the goals of treatment. It is essential that each group member develop a personal rationale for dance therapy with help from the leader as well as other group members.

It is common for borderline patients to come to treatment with a host of issues that require attention: disgust toward the body, the desire to exist without a body, a sense of being unable to move, fears about physical and emotional closeness, and extreme discomfort with angry and/or sexual feelings. Patients often say they want to find alternate ways of managing psychic numbness and dissociation. They also want to replace self-mutilation and other destructive acts with more adaptive behaviors.

A major goal in this work is to help individuals develop the capacity to create dances that are both satisfying and meaningful. Such dances are based on forms of improvisation that help individuals work spontaneously with their inner conflicts. Building a patient's capacity to tolerate the flow of internal phenomena, which are the raw materials of dance, is itself an ego-building process. The repeated reinvestment of thoughts, feelings, and sensations into dance improvisations requires tolerance for ambiguity and frustration.

Dance improvisation can move the dancer from the immediacy of feeling and sensation to symbolic expression. For example, having a tantrum is not a dance, but dancing about a tantrum is a dance. It is a creative and symbolic transformation of the feelings expressed in a tantrum. When they dance, these patients are often overwhelmed by their impulses. The ideal course of treatment then involves a gradual progression toward the inclusion of chaotic aspects of psychic life into the domain of symbolization. It can be useful for the therapist to suggest to impulsive patients to "try to maintain an observing sense of yourself while you are moving." In this light, the dancer can be thought of as psychically separate *from* but interacting *with* her dance. Such a suggestion may be offered to guide the patient in the direction of an increasing capacity for self-reflection and self-control.

The dance therapist is first faced with the task of creating a cohesive and cooperative group—a group in which authority issues and threats to self-cohesion could easily obstruct a smooth development. Fears related to coercion and humiliation can cause members to avoid engaging in movement. For these reasons, group members require a high degree of structure in the early stages. The ground rules of treatment need to be made clear.

Patients need continual reassurance that the pace will allow for individual variations in timing, intensity of expression, and need for structure. Warm-up exercises focus on remediative work that addresses members' physical and emotional needs. For example, exercises may focus on breathing, groundedness, fluidity, and the organization of movement sequences. The criteria for a successful warm-up is that members are ready to improvise. The therapist knows this by observing each person's degree of concentration and investment in the warm-up. Clarity of movement may indicate an understanding of the instructions whereas a vague series of motions or a distracted facial expression convey that the patient may not be genuinely engaged.

The borderline patients' ability to tolerate freedom of movement is limited. For this reason it is important to provide movement suggestions or formats that combine a balance of structure and freedom. The following is an example of a format that addresses a frequent theme.

Patients often speak of "losing" themselves when they dance in dyads. A common complaint is that one dancer ends up copying her partner's movements and feeling coerced. The therapist can translate this problem of autonomy into movement terms with the following: "Find a way to continue your movement while noticing your partner's dance. See if you wish to make one change while interacting with your partner. Experiment by going back and forth between your movements and incorporating your partner's dance."

The Role of the Dance Therapist

The therapist's role involves a variety of functions, many of which are basic to most forms of psychotherapy. She observes, evaluates, formulates, and makes trial verbal interventions. The phenomenon of a therapist who moves presents a number of unique issues, however. The dance therapist is in a role of high visibility in which her own inner reactions and attitudes can be revealed in her movement behavior. She makes interventions on a movement level and teaches improvisation through demonstration. She may also contribute certain movement or emotional themes to amplify what she perceives as the group's dynamics and emotions.

As in every form of therapy, patients bring significant aspects of past relationships into the group. Old conflicts are represented in the present situation with an emotional immediacy. The therapist's role is always to understand the meaning of the patients' reactions in the context of their pasts. This does not necessarily mean that everything is interpreted. Instead, the therapist chooses interventions that enhance the integration of movement behavior and psychological development—aware that such integration can facilitate the patient's insight.

A group of female patients had difficulty acknowledging feelings of possessiveness toward the therapist and envy of each other. One patient daringly danced out the ruthlessness she felt in her desire to own the therapist and her self-hatred about this impulse. Putting words to her dance, she said, "I can't have me if I don't have you!" In response group members developed their own dances of invidious longing and self-contempt. When it was the therapist's turn to improvise, she reflected the movement themes she had seen, but also grounded herself with soothing movements and said, "hurting but holding my own." The patients recognized that the therapist had received their message, and presented a solution that had not occurred to them—the possibility of finding stability even in the face of emotional pain. The capacity to provide self-comfort represents the internalization of a nurturing figure.

Borderline patients with a traumatic history may need an extraordinary amount of reassurance and support in their attempts to experience and reintegrate aspects of the past. For this reason, some modification in treatment may be warranted. Improvisations about traumatic experiences must allow for the slow integration and consolidation of previously disavowed aspects of the self. Such improvisations are often most productive if the time allotted is brief and the patient feels in control of the structure and depth of the experience. Giving individuals control of the time factor reduces their anxiety, which stems from the fear of retraumatization. A modest pace, with episodes of short improvisation, discussion, group sharing, and a return to improvisation is recommended.

Individuals need the safety of a "facilitating environment" (Winnicott, 1971) in order to develop a bodily sense of vitality and the capacity to play. This often requires the presence of a warm, empathic therapist. The patient's idealization of the therapist may not be pathological but well within the course of normal development (Kohut, 1977; Stern, 1985). As has been stated previously, movement is so close to the impulses that it can bring about further loss of control. A selfobject transference with the therapist can function as a source of stabilization against fragmentation. The borderline patient's condition, which often includes excessive aggression, requires special consideration. Although it may at times be optimal to confront a patient's resistance or acting out behavior in verbal therapy, the same approach will not necessarily work in dance therapy, where an individual must feel safe in order to move.

Countertransference reactions include the entire range of the therapist's responses to the patient. Because of the intense relationship these individuals form with the therapist, countertransference may be evoked frequently and suddenly and must be understood in order to be used effectively in treatment. Borderline patients depend on the group leader to contain their movement and their impulses. Although the therapist undergoes her own pressures during the course of any group, she strives to maintain neutrality. The therapist attempts to create a nonjudgmental environment in which all aspects of the member's difficulties can be expressed. However the nature of patient's problems will almost inevitably bring up complex personal issues for the therapist.

For example, prior to a particular session the therapist had a distinct feeling of dread before entering the treatment room. Afterward she recalled seeing all the faces turn as she took her place among the group. The group began with each member doing a brief improvisation. As the leader took her turn, she was surprised to find herself plucking imaginary sticky material off her arms. Her association, which she did not share with the patients, was that she was removing leeches from her body. Her reaction to the aggressive and clinging nature of the group members was expressed in this spontaneous movement image and gave her an immediate insight into how she experienced the group that day.

Conclusions

The vignettes presented in this chapter took place in a day treatment center that had an emphasis on therapeutic community. One advantage of this setting was the opportunity for the dance therapist to function in a variety of therapeutic roles. This offered an enriched perspective on the patients, and the patients benefited from being seen from several vantage points by the same therapist. It may be that such a situation can help borderline patients develop a more coherent and consistent sense of self and others.

It cannot be overemphasized that a treatment using body movement as an entry into inner life is different than one that enters through the verbal sphere. It is the authors' belief that the change process in therapy is based on the development of insight. Insight is a complex human phenomenon that necessarily affects cognition, affect, and behavior simultaneously. Insight can be initiated from many directions. In dance therapy, access to the individual's psychic world is through movement. New movement behavior can promote insight. Similarly, insight can promote new behavior. When movement is utilized to get at the richness of human experience the aim is for the total integration of the individual.

It is impressive how consistently patients express a desire not to surrender to the constrictions of their psychopathology. Borderline patients are constantly involved in a struggle to maintain daily functioning, to endure emotional suffering, and to resist suicide. Inhibitions and deficits in the domains of sexuality, playfulness, assertiveness, and creativity restrict their pleasure in the present and, more importantly, threaten their hope for a better future. It seems essential to return to the realm of the body in order to provide a restitutive experience and to help generate and maintain a vital sense of aliveness. This vitality can be used to fuel the psychic functions of stabilization and self-soothing. This in turn enhances the cohesion and continuity of the developing sense of self.

5

Multiple Personality Disorder: A Group Movement Therapy Approach

Edith Z. Baum

Multiple personality disorder (MPD)* is a complex, chronic dissociative disorder characterized by disturbances of memory and identity (Nemiah, 1980; Kluft, 1987). As a defensive response to trauma, MPD is almost invariably a result of overwhelming childhood experiences (Putnam, Guroff, Silberman, Barban, & Post , 1984; Spiegel, 1984). Traumatized individuals dissociate from the pain by creating both "alter" personalities and alternative "realities." From a movement perspective, MPD patients may be understood to cut themselves off from their feelings by armoring their bodies. In this way they separate their physical and psychological selves (Baum, 1993).

Dissociative and Multiple Personality Disorder

Psychiatric interest in dissociation began with the work of Pierre Janet (1859–1947). Janet treated patients who suffered from amnesias, psychogenic fugues, successive existences or altered states, and conversion symptoms.[1] His studies led him to postulate that dissociative disturbances originated with traumatic experiences in early childhood. Further, he believed treatment could alle-

---

*Now termed Dissociative Identity Disorder in DSM IV (1994)

viate symptoms by bringing split-off feelings and memories into awareness (Putnam, 1989).

Interest in dissociation has gained momentum as the result of several factors. Dissociative disorders, such as MPD, were given a more prominent position in the 1980 edition of the *Diagnostic and Statistical Manual of Mental Disorders* (DSM-III) than they had in previous editions. The women's movement brought attention to the previously unrecognized frequency of abuse directed at children and women. Clinicians started to listen more carefully to accounts of childhood sexual abuse instead of discounting them as fantasies (Kramer, 1991). Following the Vietnam war, Post–traumatic Stress Disorder (PTSD), which contains dissociative characteristics, gained acceptance in the therapeutic milieu (Kluft, 1991) and brought attention to the various consequences of severe trauma.

Dissociation is defined as the separation of an idea or thought process from the main stream of consciousness (Braun, 1988a, 1988b). It can be measured on a continuum, varying from the common, hypnotic-like trance one may experience driving on a highway to the maladaptive and pathological trance-state incurred by the MPD patient. In the MPD patient, as stated above, there is a disruption in memory and identity. This complex phenomenon can be conceptualized according to Braun's (1988a, 1988b) "BASK" model, an acronym that represents behavior, affect, sensation, and knowledge. Braun describes these four as parallel processes that function over time. Dissociation can occur in any one or more of these processes. It is the therapist's aim to help the patient bring the dissociated experience to light and make it congruent with the individual's total functioning, that is, the BASK dimensions. In other words, the goal is restoration of the dissociated aspects of the individual to the ongoing flow of consciousness.

The BASK model can be used to differentiate various forms of dissociation. For example, in sleepwalking, behavior is ongoing, but out of awareness. Affect and knowledge are absent, although sensation is more or less continuous. This can be contrasted to a hypnotically induced surgical anesthesia in which affect and sensation are separated from the individual's actions and knowledge. Likewise, an MPD patient may have knowledge of a significant event in his past and be able to report the facts, but lack the affect and sensation that commonly accompany an important memory.

For example, a behavioral clue to an MPD patient's dissociation occurred when, after a sudden loud noise, she was found rocking and mutely staring into space. The patient had previously been diagnosed as suffering from right-sided migraine headaches that were accompanied by abnormal redness on the right temple. When the patient was able to speak, she complained of a severe right-sided headache and said she was terrified by the noise. The following story was pieced together from various alters.

When the patient was 5 years old, her father and his brother got into a fight in her home. Frightened, she hid under the basement stairs. Soon afterward, her father and uncle came tumbling down the stairs and landed near her hiding place. Her father picked up a gun and shot her uncle, killing him. The patient came out of hiding. Her father grabbed her and put the still hot gun to her temple. Clicking the trigger, he threatened her into keeping his secret.

This incident was so traumatic that polyfragmentation occurred and the trauma was frozen in time. Different aspects of the incident were kept separate via multiple dissociations. For example, one part of the self rocked; other parts knew about the fighting, hiding, and gunshots. When the incident was finally pieced together, the host personality sensed relief. The patient's headaches, which had been caused by the rapid switching between fragments, dissipated. Intrapsychic association stimulated by the loud noise had reactivated the initial trauma. The rocking behavior was a repetition of the comforting movement of the frightened little girl hiding under the stairs. The red temple was a psychophysiological memory of where her father had pressed the gun to her head (Braun, 1988a, 1988b).

Multiple Personality Disorder is characterized by dramatic transformations of self. Such changes occur when separate and autonomous altered states of consciousness have successive control of behavior. Outwardly, these alterations vary from barely observable changes, such as slight muscle movements around the mouth, to more extreme, dramatic shifts.

According to the 1987 revised edition of the Diagnostic and Statistical Manual of Mental Disorders, the diagnostic criteria for MPD consist of:

1. The existence within the person of two or more distinct personalities or personality states, each with its own relatively enduring pattern of perceiving, relating to, and thinking about the environment and self.

2. At least two of these personalities or personality states recurrently take full control of the person's behavior (APA, 1987, p. 272).

Altered states, or personalities, may differ in age, gender, race, religion, and sexual orientation. In addition, they may present themselves as nonhuman: as deities, demons, angels, or animals. Different personalities may have distinct allergic reactions or may vary in their response to medication and eyeglass prescriptions. Other differences may occur in handedness, handwriting, voice, vocabulary, accents, speech patterns, and languages (Kluft, 1991).

Presenting MPD symptoms range from depression, suicide attempts, panic attacks, phobias, substance abuse, eating disorders, psychoses (which include auditory and visual hallucinations), migraines, obsessive compulsions and rituals. It is easy to understand why such patients often remain in the mental health system for many years before they are properly diagnosed. Once properly diagnosed, however, treatment is manageable even though the healing process is often fraught with resistance and difficulty.

MPD Patients in Therapy Groups

For MPD patients who are often disconnected from their traumatic experiences, verbal psychotherapy, the traditional treatment of choice, progresses more effectively in conjunction with nonverbal modalities (Kluft, 1984a, 1988b). The therapeutic process and techniques involved in interdisciplinary collaboration, such as the use of one modality to negotiate an impasse in another, have been well documented (Baum, Kluft, & Reed, 1984; Kluft, 1993; Levy, 1979, 1992). Art and movement facilitate the uncovering of material, enhance the integrative process, and afford the patient an opportunity to participate in the milieu. Working individually or in groups, MPD patients learn to express feelings through words and movements, thereby weaving together the physical and psychological aspects of themselves. While individual verbal therapy concentrates on the resolution of internal conflicts, a small therapy group helps the patient understand the concept of self in the world. "Group therapy presents an opportunity for the MPD patient to participate in a sense of togetherness, with other humans in a social context" (Caul, Sachs, & Braun, 1986, p. 147).

Although MPD patients often do poorly in groups with a diverse psychiatric population (Caul, 1984; Caul, et al., 1986; Coons & Bradley, 1985; Kluft, 1984a, 1984b), with adequate structure, a group devoted solely to MPD patients provides a useful healing experience. Based on this concept, in the summer of 1989 the Institute of the Pennsylvania Hospital opened a 13-bed dissociative disorder unit. Today the hospital is recognized for its pioneering work with MPD patients. Movement therapy, seen as a means to decrease isolation and encourage interrelatedness among MPD patients, is an integral part of the treatment. Movement has been found to be particularly helpful in bringing to awareness traumatic material that needs to be identified, expressed, and worked through in individual therapy. Likewise, thoughts and feelings first recognized in a verbal session can then be explored in movement. Such synergy facilitates increased connections across the BASK dimensions and encourages integration.

As stated above, MPD patients respond to trauma by disconnecting from their feelings. The original trauma, which created a sense of powerlessness, also produced feelings of betrayal, guilt, rage, and depression. Reexperiencing the trauma can be equally overwhelming and can further the patient's denial and emotional numbing (Horowitz, Wilmer, Kaltreider, & Alvarez, 1980). MPD patients are often reluctant to move freely because they fear arousing unconscious material that will lead them to lose control. They keep a cautious watch against triggering memories. MPD patients seem to intuitively appreciate the evocative power of movement and its ability to reconnect them to their pasts (Baum, 1991). Painful memories, however, must be faced, and worked through, if healing is to occur (E.S. Kluft, 1993).

Interventions

Two movement therapy groups for MPD patients were formed on the Dissociative Disorder Unit at the Institute. Each group, consisting of seven to eight female patients, met biweekly for 1-hour sessions. The groups had no male members as none had been admitted to the unit.

A session commonly begins with group members sitting in a circle of chairs. The group decides on the choice of music, and members often bring their own tapes or records. Each person takes a turn initiating warm-up movements of a particular body part. During this period, the therapist has an opportunity to assess the mood of each member, gathering information that can later be developed in the session.

At the end of the warm-up, the group stands. The therapist may begin by reflecting, through her own movements, a member's conscious or unconscious expression. The group replicates the leader's movement, trying to identify with the feelings expressed. Eventually, each member is encouraged to initiate an expressive movement.

Establishing Trust Through Kinesthetic Empathy

Securing trust is the initial building block on which all else is based. With this particular population, trust needs to be reestablished on a continuous basis. It is perhaps the key issue and most difficult aspect of treatment.

Kinesthetic empathy is expressed through the therapist's sensitive replication of the patient's movement behavior. This empathic response from the therapist helps to develop trust and begin the formation of a therapeutic alliance. As trust increases, patients find it easier to express repressed emotions and images. When this process takes place safely, the patients are free to express the underlying truth of their personal histories through their movements.

Negotiating Social Interaction

Within the group setting, participants learn how their own movement affects others and how they react to others' movement. From this, patients can begin to identify dysfunctional styles of interaction and to practice alternative behaviors. For example, one self-absorbed patient, Alease, arrived in an extremely angry state. When it was her turn to initiate movement, she picked up a chair, placing it in front of her, and kicked it across the room. Although this behavior frightened everyone in the group, one patient, Jane, had a particularly strong reaction. In response to Alease's behavior, Jane ran to a corner of the room, switched to a trembling child alter, and remained crouched on the floor until one of the leaders could get the child alter to "step back" and assure Jane that it was safe to return. The chair was removed and Alease was asked to find a more appropriate way to express her rage. She was suddenly immobilized by the recognition that her impulsive behavior had frightened others. Encouraging Alease to join them, some of the group members began to move together. She made meager attempts to follow the movement and later apologized to the group for frightening them.

Group cohesiveness develops gradually as members come to appreciate the common bonds of their disorder. Trust initially placed in the therapist is extended to group members as they move together. When, in the middle of a session, one patient suddenly responds to inner stimuli or an alter initiates a new movement pattern, group members can embody the specific dynamic qualities. During the discussion that follows the movement, patients are encouraged to provide support and feedback to one another. The MPD patients thus serve as auxiliary observing egos for one another even though their own fragmentation, amnesia, and distorted perceptions of self often limit their capacity to do this for themselves.

Eliciting Expressive Movement and Traumatic Material

It is necessary that patients be encouraged to identify and express feelings without hurting themselves or others. Acting out needs to be contained. Once clear and supportive boundaries have been established and an environment for open feedback has been encouraged, patients can begin to learn new skills in managing the rages common to individuals with MPD.

An example of eliciting expressive movement occurred when Randy, a relative newcomer to the group, fell to the floor in reaction to another group member's powerful expression of anger. Randy told the group that as a child she had never been allowed to express her feelings. At the next session, she began to move gently and rhythmically and then began to stamp her feet. Next, she bent her knees and leaned backward and switched to another personality, a male alter. She brought her arm close to her side, and quickly thrust it outward and lunged forward. Her whole body began to tremble and she retreated to a chair. The therapist suggested that the angry male alter step back and that Randy come forward. After a moment, Randy returned but was aware of what had happened and stated that she would have to punish herself for getting angry. The individual who had abused Randy as a child had not allowed her any display of anger. This inhibition had prevented Randy from expressing herself for many years. Her expression of rage came about as a result of the therapist's support ("all parts of the mind are welcome here"), and her observation of a peer taking similar risks.

Reflecting another's movements can help a patient get in touch with her own repressed material and can cause spontaneous abreaction. Abreaction is an emotional release or discharge that accompanies the recollection of a painful, previously repressed experience. Positive therapeutic effect occurs as emotions are discharged and insight is established.

For example, Maya arrived at the movement group looking extremely anxious. She had just returned from a session with her doctor. During the warm-up she appeared preoccupied and had difficulty following other's movements. It was not until a peer suddenly began to initiate strong punches that Maya became involved. She replicated the angry movements, something she had never done before. As she punched, her eyes filled with terror. She clutched her throat, gasping that she had asthma and couldn't breathe. Maya was suddenly experiencing a spontaneous abreaction. During this she recovered a memory of having been sexually abused. While Maya punched at the air, she relived the traumatic experience. Behavior and sensation suddenly reassociated with affect and knowledge. The behavior was punching, the affect was rage and terror, the sensation was loss of breath, and the knowledge was the memory of the abuse.

As in the above example, movement stimulates the sensory motor components of repressed memories (the sensation and behavior dimensions of BASK). At the same time, increasing awareness of one's moving body supports the mastery of overwhelming affect. Although the fluid nature of movement stimulates both fear of disorganization and loss of control, it also has the potential for integration of feeling, thought, and action. Alters emerge, making themselves known by movement patterns that tell different pieces of their stories. The validation received from the group's replication of these patterns can empower the patient regardless of which alter is moving. Images that spontaneously emerge during the group join with kinesthetic sensation and slowly become connected to memories. This connectedness promotes a sense of personal autonomy and a gradual sense of integration. As one patient remarked, "This group is helpful because as I am able to reexperience the feelings that have been buried, I am able to begin to feel whole, rather than fractured into many pieces."

The following example illustrates abreaction in one individual triggered by another individual's expression. Mary seemed depressed when she arrived. She initiated movement to a piece of dirge-like music she had brought to the session. As the music played, Mary slowly lowered her body until her knees touched the floor, she curled her head down, her chin touched her chest and her hands covered her head. She remained motionless and then slowly rocked from side to side. Other group members followed her movement.

Lee, another member of the group, tilted her upper body to one side until she slid onto her hip. Her face was contorted and she appeared dissociated. Dragging one leg, she began to move and made a deep moaning sound. The other patients were so frightened by Lee they had to be taken temporarily outside the movement room. Meanwhile, the therapist stooped down to Lee and told her she was safe. Lee reached up and took the therapist's hand and drew close. She continued moaning and her body trembled. She reached up to her lips, her head thrown back. She touched her lips and tried to speak. The therapist held her, reassuring her that she was safe.

After several minutes, in order to bring Lee into the present, the therapist asked her what year it was and where she was. She said, "1992" and after a short pause, "We're in the movement room." Sobbing, she said that it felt as if her lips had been sewn together when she was a child. She continued to sob, but couldn't say more about the sensation. After this experience her breathing became calmer and deeper.

The group came back together in a circle to process what had happened. Mary, the patient whose movement triggered Lee's abreaction, felt responsible for upsetting Lee. Lee reassured her, telling her that she had done nothing wrong. She said that what Mary expressed moved her so deeply that it had gotten her in touch with her own buried pain. She explained that the knot in her stomach, which had been there for 20 years, now felt better, like something had been released.

Although one part of Lee relived a traumatic experience, another part was, at the same time, able to view it from the present. The session proved to be significant to her in the recovery and integration of traumatic memories. She was able to reassociate sensation (knot in her stomach), affect, and behavior (her experience of pain), with the recollection of a traumatic event (alleged experience of her lips being sewn). Her subsequent calmness and concern for the other patients demonstrated a step forward toward a coherent self.

Conclusions

Movement focuses on the body and body memory. Since the MPD patient has often been abused, the use of expressive movement can be extremely provocative and so must be used cautiously. Because of their painful memories, MPD patients divide their consciousness and create alternate personalities. By granting these alters permission to form and shape their experience, both in movement and words, MPD patients are given an opportunity to express themselves and their stories. In this process MPD patients are facilitated in the integration of disowned aspects of themselves and the reunification of the behavioral, affective, sensory, and cognitive components of their past.

6

Walls of Addiction

M. Barbara Murray-Lane

Over the last 20 years, the number of women addicted to drugs and alcohol has increased dramatically. Until the past decade, the substance abuse field has unfortunately focused research, education, prevention, and treatment primarily on men. As the statistics climb, the field is challenged to address the pressing and unique issues of the chemically dependent woman.

An Overview of the Literature

Historically, gender has been viewed as irrelevant to an understanding of chemical dependency. Recent literature clearly indicates that chemical dependency affects women differently from men in important ways, however. Women drink at an earlier age, for example, and account for half of all alcohol drinkers (Peluso & Peluso, 1988). In addition, from the onset of drinking, the stages of alcoholism progress at a more rapid rate for women than men (Mendelson & Mello, 1985). In one study on cirrhosis of the liver, although the male mortality rate was 11 times higher than that of the general population, the rate for women was 25 times higher (Peluso & Peluso, 1988).

The data for women are alarming. Two million women are addicted to prescription drugs. A 1984 national survey of drug use among high school seniors found that three times as many female students as males used diet pills. In women over 65, three times as many use sedatives and antidepressants than do their male counterparts. In 1978, 12 million women had taken stimulants, outnumbering men two to one. Heroin addiction is increasing at a faster rate for women than for men and twice as many women as men are admitted to hospital emergency rooms for drug overdose (Peluso, et al., 1988).

In addition to these disturbing findings, women also bring gender-specific issues to treatment. More than half of all chemically dependent women are survivors of incest, molestation, and/or sexual assault (Covington, 1985). Many are promiscuous, have been sexually assaulted, or have engaged in prostitution while under the influence. Others use chemicals to blunt the painful memories of childhood abuse. Some view being a woman in itself as a painful and defective burden. Bradshaw (1988) believes that at the core of addictive behaviors is a condition he calls "toxic shame," the sense of experiencing oneself as flawed and defective as a person. Women experience a greater sense of shame and social stigma about their chemical dependence than do men, and suffer, as well, from more intense feelings of self-hatred and mistrust (Morrison, 1986). Babcock and Connor (1981) state that women internalize a greater negative self-image due to their alcoholism, bringing an increased burden of guilt and low self-esteem to treatment. Fuhlrodt (1990) finds that women are more able than men to identify the painful causes of their addiction. In addition, they blame themselves for their disease regardless of their life situations. They are also secretive about their addiction, which creates a vicious cycle.

Chemically dependent women also seem to struggle with a more impenetrable denial system. Social stigma, secrecy, and family's minimizations serve to protect and fortify this denial. This results in the development of two distinct parts of the woman, the addicted and the healthy part (Kasl, 1989). Each denies the existence of the other. As the addiction gains control, the denial system becomes increasingly rigid. The healthy side of the addict becomes overwhelmed and, eventually, as the disease progresses, the consequences of the addiction are minimized.

The literature further suggests that chemically dependent women benefit from gender-specific treatment (Morrison, 1986). In groups with men, women often take on the role of facilitator and nurturer, and thus avoid their own problems. Participation in an all-female group allows women to address issues they might not otherwise discuss, partially due to the roles typically assigned to women by men. Babcock and Connor (1981) suggest that an all-women's group be led by female therapists in order to provide role modeling and promote assertiveness.

Treatment Setting

The program provides intensive treatment for women through either a 28-day inpatient or a 6-week outpatient program. The staff of women includes a social worker, family and marriage therapist, nurse, creative-arts therapists, residential counselors, and an aerobic instructor. The program is tightly structured with a daily educational component, a variety of therapy groups, an exercise and relaxation program, assertiveness training, self-esteem groups, and nightly Alcoholics Anonymous and Narcotics Anonymous meetings. Dance/movement therapy meets three times a week for an hour and is mandatory. The session size varies but averages about eight members. Verbal processing usually begins and ends each session.

The Expression of Shame

Prior to the session, this group of three women had attended a seminar on the relationship between feelings of shame and addiction. All of the women had been troubled by the discussion of shame. In a joint decision with the therapist, the women decided to continue exploring the theme of shame through expressive movement.

At the therapist's suggestion, each woman was given time to develop four movement actions that reflected her feelings, and then was asked to share with the group her completed movement sequence. Sequences were then repeated with word associations. Finally, the members were told they could add or change any part of their sequence.

Mary

Mary is a tall white woman in her late 20's. Divorced with a young daughter, before treatment she had maintained a full-time job with a city government. She reported a long history of substance abuse beginning in early adolescence. In her first session, she had spoken of hating her body and her feelings and not wanting to be in the group. She became easily frustrated and utilized anger to distance the therapist and her peers.

Her movement sequence and word associations were as follows: Mary swung her arms and skipped toward the group; she smiled and said, "happy." Next, still facing the group, with eyes downcast, she touched her breasts and genitals roughly, began to cry and said, "disgust." Then Mary punched the air and gestured obscenely. She continued crying and shouted, "anger!" In the last movement Mary dropped her head, turned away from the group with her arms across her chest, and tearfully whispered, "shame."

After her initial demonstration, Mary added one change to the end of her sequence. She turned toward the group, her arms remained across her chest. She lifted her eyes to meet her peers and repeated, "shame."

In the discussion at the end of the session, Mary revealed to the group that she had been sexually abused in childhood. She recognized the shame and disgust she felt for her body. Her first movement sequence seemed to show a happy young girl. Her shame is indicated in her second movement by the lack of eye contact and the rough way she touched herself. Mary's feelings of anger and shame had become chronic but mood-altering substances had kept the feelings at bay. Despite the drugs, her secrets haunted her. She began to wonder if her compulsive eating and aggressive behaviors were a defense. Mary's final movement sequence portrayed that her secrets included sadness. She told the group that this was the first time she was able to talk about the past.

Doris

Doris is a heavyset black woman in her late 60's. Married and a homemaker with three grown sons, she had been drinking for most of her adult life and, as a result, had sustained much physical deterioration. She had had multiple car accidents while intoxicated. Her family always minimized and rationalized the extent of Doris' drinking. Up until this session, Doris had presented herself as passive and compliant. She talked little, had difficulty relating to the other women and, overall, was isolated and withdrawn.

In this session, of her own initiative, she spoke openly of her alcoholism and her humiliation. Her movement sequence was made up of only three actions. First, Doris looked around the room, as if to see if someone was watching, she lowered her head, slumped, and passively motioned as if drinking. She said quietly, "secret." Then she turned quickly away from the group, ran to a corner of the room and said, "runaway." Doris remained in the corner with her back to the group and, cowering, said "shame." She added one movement to the end of her sequence. She returned to the group, faced her peers with some assertion and weight in her posture, made eye contact and said, "sober."

In the discussion, Doris continued to speak of her feelings. She said she was embarrassed and self-conscious because of the "secret." This feeling can be noted in Doris's first movement sequence with lowered head and slumped posture. The power of her secret fueled her discomfort with herself, as shown in the movements that followed. Doris's sense of herself had been diminished each time she drank and lost control, and had been compounded when her family rescued her from the aftermath of her drinking. She connected this to her denial and the difficulty she had accepting her disease. The use of more assertive movements as in the last sequence, enabled Doris to experience herself differently. This allowed her, for the moment, to break through her denial, connect to her contemporaries and develop a sense of hope.

Christine

Christine, a frail woman in her mid-30's, had been smoking, snorting, and shooting one type of drug or another for 20 years. She had recently lost her husband, job, and home due to her addiction. She also had been working as a prostitute to support her habit. In previous sessions she had said she enjoyed and felt comfortable moving. She had been expressive in the group, exhibiting a positive connection and an eagerness to utilize the group for self-discovery.

In her first movement Christine faced the group smiling and began to skip in a circle and sing softly to herself. She sang, "innocent." Then she began to jerk her body in many directions as if pulled by invisible ropes. The movements were initially slow and appeared painful. The movements became quicker as if now she was being pushed in many directions. She cried, "secrets." Next, Christine began to whirl round and round, at first in a controlled and slow fashion and then faster and faster until she appeared out of control. She yelled, "drugs." Finally, she fell to the floor in a ball and sobbed. Later she labeled this, "shame!" At the end of this sequence, Christine added one last movement. She lifted herself up from the floor and crawled forward; she said, "toward the light."

Like Mary, Christine's initial movement sequence depicted a time in her past when she had been confident and carefree. In the discussion, Christine said she had always felt she had lost something, which in turn resulted in a sense of herself as defective and empty. As a consequence, her body had become something to torment and abuse with drugs and sex. The second movement sequence demonstrated the painful and destructive place secrets had in her life, and the next sequence showed how Christine used drugs to control and silence the secrets. In the discussion, she connected her addiction to heroin, and her prostitution to an effort to fill the emptiness she experienced. Childhood sexual abuse, drug addiction, prostitution, loss of husband and job created profound feelings of despair. The final movement sequence indicated some of what she had learned during her hospitalization—the recognition of her powerlessness over her pain, and her need to reach beyond herself to overcome her addictions.

The suggestion to the group to develop movement sequences related to the topic of shame prompted personal insight. The women used the movement to trace the progression of their self-rejection and hatred. Movement also facilitated the development of alternative choices. Each woman acknowledged a secret that was core to the rejection of herself. Because of the intense nature of the women's experiences at the hospital, defenses were often penetrated quickly, as shown above and in the next example.

Walls of Defense

The group consisted of eight women; five were alcoholic and three drug addicted. They ranged in age from 26 to 60, with a mixture of African Americans, Caucasians, and Hispanics. The group had been working together intensely for 2 weeks without admissions or discharges, which allowed for in-depth exploration.

Prior to the session, the women had attended an educational workshop on denial. This session began with a brief discussion about what they had learned. They talked about their walls, barriers, and defenses.

When the group began, the members were asked to build a wall representing the part of them that was addicted. Cardboard bricks, pillows, scarves, index cards with printed words, blankets, and masks were distributed. Without hesitation, the walls were built. Most of the women chose to make their structures on the edges of the room, thereby including the walls of the room in the design. A few remained in the center of the space. The walls were formidable; tall and enclosing with no evident doors or windows. The women assigned words to their walls such as "Back off," 'I'm fine," "I don't have a problem," "I don't need any one," and "Leave me alone." They also drew pictures of stop signs, obscene gestures, and danger warnings. Masks of roaring lions, growling tigers, angry bears, and watching owls were posted on the walls. When finished, the women became quiet. They were isolated from one another. They were then asked to place themselves in some meaningful relationship to their walls.

A pale young woman of 20 sat with her knees pressed up to her chin, arms wrapped tightly around her legs. She said "My addict side is frightened. My drinking is all I've ever known." Her wall was large and meticulous. She had spent a long time building it "just right."

A strong stout woman had built her wall tightly around herself, enclosing her body up to her nose with only her dark sunglasses peeking out. She said "I feel like this owl on my wall...always watching to see if it's safe...untrusting and paranoid."

A usually boisterous woman in her mid-50's lay wrapped in a blanket in a fetal position. Her wall covered her body. She said "I'm alone. I've got my pills and my pain. It's killing me but I don't need anyone."

The group remained like this for a long time. The therapist asked quietly if they wanted to remain behind their walls or if they wanted to make changes. With a dramatic burst of energy, three of the women jumped up and began knocking down their walls. They threw bricks, ripped papers, pulled down masks, and discarded blankets. The others moved more cautiously, enlarging their walls to include doors or windows, changing the words and symbols to reflect more inviting statements.

At this point, the group took on a life of its own with few directions. The women who had knocked down their walls came together in a circle and held hands. They stood in the middle of the room quietly. The other women watched from behind their walls. The therapist commented on the internal struggle being expressed about change and suggested testing the unfamiliar territory outside the wall by joining the circle. Slowly, and at different intervals, the women joined the circle, remained briefly, and then returned to the security of their walls. They moved back and forth, vacillating between the familiar and unfamiliar. This process continued for a long time. Eventually, the women all remained standing in the circle. They swayed ever so slightly. Then, softly at first, almost in a whisper, one woman began to recite the Lord's Prayer. The volume increased as the others joined her. The group ended at this point.

In the discussion that followed, the women identified anger, aggression, and isolation as the behavioral building blocks that shaped their denial systems. They recognized the walls as entrenched patterns; they felt they could not escape.

Anxiety and fear were experienced whenever they were asked to express the healthy side, the side that had the potential to change. Many of the women said they could not have approached such change without the support from the group. Even with support, however, it was a difficult process. They acknowledged that the addiction was both familiar and seductive and that the battle ahead would not be easy.

In the circle, they felt "safe" and "accepted." This was translated in their bodies as "connecting" and "opening." Eventually they all expressed the desire to stay connected to the circle. The movement work allowed the women in both groups to experience themselves from within, and apart from, their addiction and to take the risk of acknowledging a capacity for health.

7

Movement as Metaphor: Treating Chemical Addiction

Sherry Rose

This chapter discusses a dynamic short-term treatment approach using group dance/movement therapy to address the problem of chemical addiction. The therapy is based on the work of Edward Khantzian (1985, 1986, Khantzian, Halliday, & McAuliffe, 1990) who developed a verbal group therapy model for substance abusers. Khantzian (1985) proposes a "self-medication" hypothesis based on his understanding of the psychological vulnerabilities that predispose individuals to substance abuse. Four areas of difficulty are focused on during the treatment process: self-esteem, feelings, relationships, and self-care.

The approach discussed here reflects Khantzian's, et. al. (1990) recommendations to address the needs and issues of abusers. It emphasizes present experience while not ignoring the past, attempts to enhance awareness of self and others, provides opportunities for problem solving and decision making, and helps group members practice alternative ways of behaving and coping. These goals will be illustrated by clinical case vignettes.

Chemical Addiction

Derived from the Latin *addictus,* meaning to devote or surrender, the word "addiction" is defined in the American Heritage Dictionary as the "compulsive...need for a habit forming substance." Such substances affect consciousness, influence the user's emotions, and alter perceptions and behaviors. Tolerance of a drug often results in an abuser's need for increasing amounts of the chosen substance in order to obtain the desired effect. As substance use progresses, the drug becomes the central organizing force in an abuser's life. Individuals who are "hooked" seek to return over and over again to the source of intoxication despite adverse physical, psychological, and social consequences. Damage may involve liver disease, memory loss, depression, the inability to keep a job, frequent accidents, and family and relationship problems, including child abuse and neglect. Moreover, thinking becomes distorted so that abusers often deny their usage and its consequences even though the effects are obvious to others. Because substances differ in their specific pharmacology, the course of abuse varies. For example, crack cocaine produces a rapid progression to addiction, whereas alcohol dependency develops more slowly, sometimes taking many years.

Chemically dependent individuals bring to treatment a range of mental health problems beyond those induced by the abuse. Although chemicals themselves can induce pathological responses, many addicted individuals struggle with preexisting psychological problems (Kaufman, 1989; Khantzian, 1985; Wurmser, 1974, 1978). Levin (1991) summarizes how chemicals are used to modulate emotional pain, as well as alter feelings and perceptions of self and others.

> [They] change mood, narcotize feelings, change self-perceptions, import either oblivion or the illusion of vitality, and give hope to the hopeless, self-esteem to the self-hating and relief from psychic pain to the emotionally wounded. They give users a sense of power. Chemicals give the illusion of magically controlling reality; they allow users to feel or be whatever they wish to feel or be. (p. 195)

Thus, chemical dependency can be viewed as a misguided attempt at self-healing. The difficulty for the addict is that substances provide false solutions. The basic disturbances remain and the user is propelled into the vicious cycle of addiction.

Whatever the initial forces that bring a person to use drugs, once addiction takes hold its grip is relentless. According to some investigators, addiction is one of the most difficult behaviors to modify (Marlatt, Baer, Donovan, & Kivlahan, 1988). Despite treatment, the risk of relapse remains high, often occurring within the first year of recovery. Therefore, short-term therapy during the early phases of recovery focuses on immediate concerns of isolation, abstinence, and relapse. It also explores the core problems of character that may have contributed to the abuse. Although short-term treatment may initially engage the individual in the recovery process, it is rarely sufficient to establish a commitment to a lifetime of sobriety. Long-term, in-depth treatment is necessary to address the behavioral and psychological problems that underlie addiction.

Treatment Approach: The Use of Movement as Metaphor

It is crucial in the treatment of chemical dependency to break through the cycle of loneliness, isolation, and despair. Common to most addicts, these feelings are often too painful to articulate in words. Movement allows group members to unite around a common theme without pressing them to verbalize their pain. It encourages feelings of connectedness, belonging, and self-affirmation.

Wallace (1989) emphasizes the value of metaphoric communication in sidestepping defenses and increasing the patient's motivation to engage in long-term treatment. Dance as art or therapy enables the representation of experience through symbols. Writing about the treatment process in dance/movement therapy, Schmais (1985) states, "The metaphoric symbol can externalize the internal state" (p. 29). The therapist can use the patient's metaphors to bring to light significant personal meanings, thereby enhancing self-awareness and understanding. For example, a severely slumped body may represent depression, whereas feet that feel "glued to the floor" provide an apt metaphor for "feeling stuck" in one's life.

The therapist's interventions have greater impact when the patient's own metaphors are used as the source of communication. In a simple example, one patient, accompanying his movement with loud whirring sounds, careened wildly around the room with his arms spread out from his body. As he bumped into other patients, he declared he was a "dive bomber." I asked him to "pull up the throttle." Drawing on the patient's metaphor I confronted the impulsive behavior without provoking a defensive response.

Confrontation, emerging self-awareness, and self-disclosure can all be constant sources of anxiety and intimidation for chemical abusers. In the face of threatening feelings, addicts often need to disengage from the group or the treatment process in order to protect themselves. Using a metaphor rather than directly confronting the behavior gives patients the needed psychic distance to remain in the session (Levy, 1988; Schmais, 1985). As group members feel less threatened, they feel less need to defend. They are more able to take in new information and consider other points of view.

Chemically dependent people often feel divided within themselves and see life in extremes. It is often helpful to ask such individuals to find movements that express these contrasts. Relationships and situations are often viewed in absolute terms, as all positive or all negative. By concretizing the extremes through dance, individuals can be helped to recognize their ambivalent feelings. In one movement session, for example, the theme of "evil" emerged in the group. Patients were encouraged to create sequences of movement that reflected this idea. Steve, a sensitive young man, felt easily threatened most of the time. In response to the movement directive he placed himself in the center of the circle and began fierce, powerful slashing movements that were aimed at each member of the group. He ended by pretending to sever his arm and then stab himself in the heart. He symbolically enacted his destructive side and called the movement sequence "death dance." I suggested that he invent a contrasting "life dance." A gay but brief twirling sequence was created with another patient. When I asked if he could merge the life and death dances he agreed to try but said he could only perform them sequentially. After his new dance, it was pointed out that his life dance had lost its initial vitality and that his death dance seemed overpowering. Steve responded, "There's another person inside me; he wants to see me in pain, but he also wants me to survive."

This experience of feeling divided into parts (see Chapter 1, this volume) is not uncommon (Levy, 1979, 1988). The anxiety these inner divisions create often propel individuals to seek relief in addictive substances. The symbolic enactment of conflicting aspects of the self allows safe expression and control of intense feelings. "When internal states are made conscious through external expression they appear less ominous" (Schmais, 1985, p. 20).

Stressing the Here and Now

It is particularly important for individuals in early recovery to address their present-day problematic behaviors and interpersonal styles of relating if they are to maintain sobriety. Since behavior problems are often acted out in maladaptive movement patterns, they can be supportively confronted within the group and made available for consideration by the patient. For example, those who are impulsive, reckless, and careless in movement are helped to see parallels in their daily lives. In one session an individual's small galloping movements turned into wild gallops around the floor as he said he was a "chariot out of control." I suggested he "pull in the reins." The movement polarities of "containment" versus "running wild" were thus juxtaposed and allowed him to experience a sense of control in the moment. The ensuing group discussion focused on impulsive behaviors and on risky situations that might trigger relapse. Because body action occurs in the "here-and-now," important insights can be derived from the immediacy of the movement experience.

Identifying Emotions

Although individuals need to increase awareness and understanding of maladaptive or self-defeating behaviors, it is also important to focus on inner emotional life. Many addicted individuals seem to act without awareness of their feelings. Some withdraw from all emotional expression, others appear to overreact. In both cases there can be a lack of emotional awareness (Khantzian, 1990; Krystal, 1977, 1982).

Alexithymia refers to individuals who are unable to identify their emotions, or distinguish one feeling from another (Krystal, 1978, 1982). Instead of discrete sensations that can be identified and articulated, emotions are experienced as uncomfortable tension states and vague, confusing body sensations. There is a persistent and often frightening sense that something is wrong in the body.

When individuals are out of touch with their inner experience, difficulties in accurately understanding others is inevitable. Thus, relationships are often painful, confusing, and fraught with problems. McDougall (1991/1982) says,

> It is evident...that an inability to capture and become aware of one's own emotional experience must be accompanied by an equally great difficulty in understanding other people's emotional states and wishes. Trapped in this psychic impasse, subjects experience an overwhelming difficulty in knowing just what people mean to them and they to others. (p. 160)

Movement exaggeration can help the alexithymic individual begin to recognize and externalize feelings.

Mary had been reared by alcoholic parents. She had difficulty recognizing and identifying her feelings, especially anger. Following a particularly intense marital therapy session, Mary came to group distraught. She paced the room and stated she was tense, confused, and uncomfortable, but didn't know why. When asked to represent her feelings with spontaneous movement and sound, she made small clawing gestures and a meek noise. Unable to exaggerate her expression, Mary was encouraged to enlist the group's help. The group exaggerated her movement and sound and when asked what they felt, they said "angry." In this process Mary became aware of her hostility toward her husband and her father. The group, accurately reflecting and embellishing Mary's actions, helped her recognize and name her feelings.

Alexithymic patients often have difficulties accessing images that are usually linked to feelings. In the following vignette, a group movement improvisation helped an alexithymic individual discover personal imagery and concomitant emotions. Gary, a passive, inhibited young man, felt "dead and empty" except when talking about drugs. After the death of his father, when he was 10, he was raised by an emotionally unavailable brother. In one session, as a result of the movement warm-up, an image of "being chained" emerged. Group members were asked to explore what being chained might feel like. Gary bent forward over himself in a kneeling position. I suggested that he allow images to surface even if they were silly or embarrassing. When none appeared, he was asked to exaggerate his posture as much as possible. Gary curled more tightly inward. Finally an image emerged: "Someone is batting a ball toward me and it hit me in the face," he responded. Initially unable to recognize the batter, he was asked to look again and this time saw his older brother. "I always felt punched in the face by him," Gary said. It emerged that Gary's brother had been physically abusive. In time, identification of his fear and anger enabled Gary to recognize his patterns of retreat.

Problem Solving and Coping Styles

Individuals who abuse substances generally tend to avoid or deny life's ordinary frustrations. The ability to problem solve is critical to a sustained recovery. The vignette below demonstrates the difficulties a patient had in finding a way to get his needs met.

John, a successful artist, had a long history of heroin use. As a child he felt unwanted and abandoned. His father worked evenings and slept days, whereas his mother, a compulsive gambler, was often negligent. When asked to structure a familial interaction, he recreated patterns of relating, conspicuous in their lack of meaningful dialogue or empathic interaction. John asked me to play the role of his mother.[1] He told me that when he shook my arm in order to get his attention, I was to point angrily toward his room. When I did so, he compliantly sat down on an imaginary bed.

John's inability to assert himself and have his interpersonal needs met was also acted out with the group. His efforts to connect with the group highlighted his dysfunctional patterns of behavior. I gave John a task: to find three alternative ways to join the group. First, he passively lay on the floor outside the circle waiting to be noticed and invited in; second, he sat behind but close to another group member and waited; and, third, he abruptly jumped into the center of the circle, pushing and shoving others in his path. John had demonstrated that he had only two patterns of interaction available: the passive helpless mode, in which he was the good little boy who waited to have his needs met; or the bad, intrusive boy. A third alternative, the assertive young man, was not part of John's repertoire. In the groups that followed, John explored different ways of satisfying his needs in relation to others.

The next vignette illustrates methods geared toward improving interpersonal functioning and coping styles. An aloof young woman, Joan, presented a grandiosity that masked her need for others and her lack of control over her heroin use. She utilized self-help group slogans superficially: "I'll take one step at a time when I'm out there," she said, or "I'll just call my sponsor." However, her movement behavior consistently betrayed the incongruence of her words.

In group Joan chose to explore her recovery, an apt theme as she was to be discharged shortly. She divided the group into "good and bad guys." The "bad guys" were identified as drug dealers and active users; the "good guys" were persons in recovery. She placed each group at opposite ends of the room and declared that her goal was to get past the bad guys in order to reach the good ones on the other side. She told the bad guys to tempt her with drugs and find ways to block her access to the other side of the room. The good guys beckoned: "Come, Joan, come to us, you can make it!" But Joan, instead of moving down the room to the good guys, paced back and forth in front of the bad guys shaking her head and arms, repeating "no, no." In spite of her efforts, Joan became embroiled with the bad guys and lost sight of her goal. When I asked her what she was doing, she said: "I'm saying no to drugs." Joan was not conscious of the futility of her efforts. Asked if she could find another way to say "no," Joan backed away from the bad guys and ended up against the wall. The group then suggested that Joan try to use her strength to push the bad guys away. She was able to push but only with the support of the other group members. As she became aware of her helplessness, she began to cry. Joan's dramatic enactment highlighted how her false posturing kept others at a distance and hid her longing for nurturance, help, and support. The movement sequence revealed the discrepancies in Joan's self-presentation. In the past, it was these discrepancies that had led to her relapses.

Self-Help Groups

Dance/movement therapy can be used to reinforce the 12-step concepts of such groups as Alcoholics Anonymous or Narcotics Anonymous. Their slogans, such as "Surrendering," "One day at a time," or "One step at a time" suggest adaptive coping responses to stressful situations and behavioral changes necessary to achieve and maintain sobriety. However, addicts are impulsive individuals for whom taking "one step at a time" is virtually unfathomable. Unaccustomed to dealing with frustration of any kind, they lack the patience to accept recovery as a process that requires time and sustained commitment. In one session a member described his relapse as "skipping steps in my recovery" and "slip slidin' away." I suggested he find a way to represent these feelings. He explored a variety of movements that included slow baby steps, quick large steps, and slippery, unstable steps. These movements exposed his conflicted desire for change and his reluctance to face the slow process of recovery. This realization is critical for patients because treatment efforts are easily sabotaged and recovery is considered a lifelong endeavor.

Conclusions

The attainment of a sober lifestyle can be considered a great achievement. Most often it takes many positive treatment experiences as well as intensive long-term aftercare that includes psychotherapy and a focus on relapse prevention, before lasting recovery is established. It is only by learning how to identify, tolerate, and process feelings and how to better manage stressful life situations that the chemically addicted person can successfully recover.

8

Confronting Co-Dependency: A Psychodramatic Movement Therapy Approach

Eileen M. Lawlor

Co-dependency, referred to as the twentieth-century condition (Cermak, 1986), has been popularized in books and periodicals, endlessly discussed on television and radio talk shows, and painfully described by participants in the anonymous fellowships of Alcoholics Anonymous (AA), Al-Anon, Adult Children of Alcoholics (ACOA), and Overeaters Anonymous (OA).[1] Co-dependency as a bona fide clinical entity is demonstrating its staying power.

Therapists and clinicians in the field are finding, however, that verbal, insight-oriented psychotherapy alone may not fully reach the deepest preverbal layers of co-dependency (Bradshaw, 1990; Whitfield, 1987). Similarly, repeated cathartic self-disclosure at 12-step meetings, while therapeutic, may not necessarily ensure that deep personal change is taking place (Smith, 1988; Wegscheider-Cruse & Cruse, 1990). Therefore, creative treatment opportunities that are designed to respond to the developmental needs of this population are necessary. The following chapter describes a psychodramatic movement-therapy approach to the treatment of co-dependency.

Co-Dependency

Following the 1989 First National Conference on Co-Dependency, an official definition was accepted: Co-dependency is the pattern of dependency on compulsive behaviors and approval-seeking in an attempt to gain safety, identity, and self-worth (Wegscheider-Cruse & Cruse, 1990).

The co-dependent is born into a family system where active addiction or another major dysfunction dominates the lives of its members. As a child, the co-dependent survives the frustration of unmet dependency needs by attempting to nurture others and, in this way, ameliorate the problems of everyone in the family. In order to do so, the child denies his or her own needs. Because of the pervasive difficulties in these families, there is no opportunity for the child's own separate and distinct development. Instead, by adapting, the child becomes dependent on the needs, wishes, hopes, and fears of the family. In other words, the child's personality is shaped co-dependently (Black, 1981; Cermak, 1985). Such home environments do not offer a place for the child to feel safe, to experience unconditional love, or to behave spontaneously.

Co-dependency can be viewed as an unconscious adaptation to a potentially threatening situation. It is an attempt to stay emotionally connected to people whose own capacity to relate to others is severely compromised. As a result of the adaptations adult co-dependents must make, they are often out of touch with their real feelings.

Developmentally, survival depends on the adequacy and willingness of the primary caregivers to deliver care. Preverbal infants appear to be able to sense major dysfunction in their caretakers and adjust to deprivation. They shut down their own expressions of need in order to please, rescue, and distract— in short, to try and "fix"—the adults on whom they should be depending. Such ingenuity represents strength that has been developed through adversity. Yet, in the case of the co-dependent, survival comes at great personal cost.

Later developmental sequences such as those associated with separation/individuation (Kohut, 1977; Mahler, Pine, & Bergman, 1975) may also be disrupted. Where this occurs, disturbances in boundary formation, discharge of feelings, and the capacity to modulate emotional closeness and distance from others are profoundly affected. The typical adult child of a dysfunctional family limps into adulthood without a solid sense of self.

Psychodramatic Movement Therapy

The multimodal psychodramatic movement therapy approach, as articulated by and demonstrated through the clinical work of Levy (1979, 1988), blends drama, graphic arts, and visual imagery with dance/movement therapy.

Movement is used to help individuals release and spontaneously explore denied thoughts and feelings. Dramatic structures are introduced to help organize the material that emerges during the spontaneous movement work. These dramatic structures are designed to help clarify the individual's underlying feelings and conflicts.

For co-dependents, a major source of conflict lies between the part of the self that has been unconsciously dedicated to adapting to the needs of others and the less developed part of the self, which holds the real, but often repressed, thoughts and feelings. This conflict expresses itself through countless daily dilemmas or inner dramas. The use of the visual arts offers another medium through which individuals can express, organize, and clarify their internal conflicts.

The therapist also assists or directs the client by employing basic techniques such as role-playing, role-reversal, and scene setting (Z.T. Moreno, 1966; J.L. Moreno & Z.T. Moreno, 1975). These methods help the client to identify, explore, and finally resolve problematic personal issues. The dramatic structures that take shape creatively within the session are the vehicles by which the client organizes, expresses, and clarifies conflicting thoughts and feelings.

This multimodal approach sets the stage for symbolic confrontation between different aspects of the individual's self and between the self and others. The dramas can represent both past and present conflicts. When introduced at key junctures in the therapeutic process, creative actions can promote reparative experiences. Adults are offered a second chance to express parts of themselves that were not permitted to emerge in childhood. This expression provides individuals with an opportunity to attend to their previously unmet developmental needs in a creative and life-enhancing way.

Case Material

The clinical examples that follow illustrate the combined use of movement, dance, drama, and imagery. In the final case the integration of the visual arts with dramatic movement is also addressed.

Because co-dependency is thought to be based on incomplete identity formation and unclear boundaries between self and others (Bradshaw 1988, 1990; Smith 1988; Subby, 1987), clinical work often centers around issues of the self and the self in relationship to others. In the vignettes that follow, simple movement experiences lead individuals to identify thoughts, feelings, and memories that might otherwise remain repressed.

Sonya: The Caretaker

Sonya, a 35-year-old registered nurse suffering from professional "burn-out," began to dance her perception of herself as a caregiver. In Martha Graham style, she contracted and expanded, grimacing and gesturing in a torturous display of emotion. Her dance seemed an endless pouring forth or giving of herself; it lacked a time for recuperation and receiving. Sonya described herself as trapped in relationship patterns in which she was always the listener, always taking care of others. Though she was able to articulate this, she had complained for weeks that she was unable to alter her habitual responses.

Believing that an exaggeration of her dance might help Sonya to gain more insight into its symbolic meaning, I moved with her, mirroring and helping her to embellish her movement sequences until she fell to the floor exhausted. Encouraged to stay with her imagery, Sonya envisioned herself as a helpless baby asleep in her crib when suddenly her mother burst into her room, roughly picked her up and took her to the kitchen where her mother began to eat frantically. Sonya's image of herself was that of a confused and upset child responding to her frantic mother by offering her comfort.

This movement experience and the accompanying imagery enabled Sonya to form a link between her early adaptation to her needy mother and a similar adaptation she had made at work. With continued use of such interventions, the co-dependent individual, as in the case of Sonya, often encounters a destructive and frightening figure from the family-of-origin. Called up symbolically through movement and imagery, a battle with this figure often begins. The struggle that ensues may take on a life and death sense of urgency. The therapist, using these methods of intervention, must be prepared to facilitate such an "encounter," as the case of Mary Ellen will illustrate.

Mary Ellen: Confronting the Need to be Seen

Mary Ellen, a verbally and intellectually well-defended 50-year-old woman, was from a multigenerational incest family. Dubbed from childhood "the smart one, the strong one, mother's right-hand girl," Mary Ellen said that she felt "anxious and scared today" because of her mother's upcoming visit to the inpatient unit. I encouraged Mary Ellen to express her feelings in movement. In response, she began to stride nervously back and forth; she appeared pressured and tense. "I'm like a caged animal," she said.

To heighten the dramatic action, and to help clarify Mary Ellen's feelings, I moved with her. By mirroring and helping her expand her movements and sounds, Mary Ellen's feelings about her mother's visit became clearer. She grew enraged and began to growl through clenched teeth. Pacing back and forth and growling were indications of her intense frustration and fury, perhaps her feelings of being controlled by her mother and by others as well. Because her pacing seemed to lead to an increased agitation, I decided to help her focus her rage outwardly. I hoped this would release her feelings in a more constructive and personally meaningful way.

I mirrored her angry stance and raised fists. Slicing the air with large arm gestures, Mary Ellen screamed, "I feel invaded, scared....I don't want to see her." Stopping abruptly, Mary Ellen stepped outside of her drama, "Why is she coming here anyway?" she screamed. I motioned to an empty chair in the corner of the room and suggested that we move toward it together. Standing in front of the empty chair, Mary Ellen was able to envision her mother. To help her confront her feelings toward her mother and focus her expression outwardly, I suggested that Mary Ellen tell her mother what she felt and what she needed from her. Her body stiffened. Looking both shocked and fearful, she physically began to retreat and shook her head "no." I continued to support her confrontation, maintaining close proximity. We joined together in deep, coordinated breaths, preparing Mary Ellen to express what she really felt toward her mother.

Finally, in a slow and deliberate voice, Mary Ellen spoke to her mother, "I want you to see me as I really am. Not as my role; not as the strong one...I need you to acknowledge my pain...I need you to...SEE ME...You really don't see me do you...I'm truly...INVISIBLE...to you."

Such a reexperience of an unmet dependency need, such as the need to be seen for who and what one really is, appears crucial to successfully overcoming co-dependency. Confrontational experiences, such as described above, can break the spell that has previously bound the co-dependent individual to self-destructive patterns.

Al: "Little Dad"

In previous groups Al had expressed sadness about the sudden loss of his father at age 11. After his father's death, Al had become "Little Dad" for his six younger brothers and had moved with his family to a crowded, dirty fifth-floor walkup.

In this session, as Al listened to another group member's graphic details of a childhood wrought with fear and deprivation, color drained from his face. His right forearm tightened across his stomach. When Al said that he felt sick to his stomach I suggested that he close his eyes and try to stay with the feeling. Al soon began to breathe deeply and his body started to tremble. His chest appeared to fill up with feeling and then slowly curved forward as he broke into full-body sobs. I encouraged him to talk about his experience.

Sobbing while rocking himself, Al recalled with terror "rats the size of cats." I adopted a synchronous rocking motion and continued. "I can't let any of my brothers see me...I'm the oldest...I have to be brave." I let Al know that I understood what a difficult task it was for him to maintain his fatherly role when underneath he was really feeling frightened and alone.

Body memory, in the form of a "sick with fear" stomach, led Al to recall the terror of "huge rats" that had invaded his home when he was a child. The sequence that occurred in the therapy group helped Al to re-member (meaning rejoin) aspects of himself, in the context of a tragic childhood. With the help of the empathic mirroring, or what J.L. Moreno (Z.T. Moreno 1966; J.L. Moreno et al., 1975), the father of psychodrama, called doubling, Al was able to uncover repressed memories that had caused him discomfort in his adult life.

Resolving Co-Dependency: A Working Case in Progress

In order for any form of therapy to succeed, the basic drive to achieve health must reside within each individual. Therapists, however, can set the stage for healing by modeling qualities of acceptance and trust, by establishing and maintaining a symbolic work space, and by fostering the notion of adventurous play. This approach does not utilize only movement and drama, it also incorporates the visual arts and other creative and playful expressions. The exact script, sequence, or particular creative medium through which important breakthroughs occur is not known until the process unfolds. "The key is to allow individuals to move from idiom to idiom in a meaningful way and the goal is to achieve a natural flow between the media forms and the client's needs" (Levy, 1988, p. 202). By empathically shaping and directing patients' use of specific media (art, drama, movement, sound), the therapist allows patients to discover their own paths, as the following discussion of Jesse illustrates.

Jesse

Her Inner Dance. Jesse, a 41-year-old author and illustrator of children's books, entered weekly individual outpatient therapy because of severe and deepening depression and an overwhelming urge to "get in the car and drive away...forever!" Although seen by others as talented and competent, Jesse saw her life as an empty trap and hoped that a dead tree that she walked beneath each day in her yard would "just give way," and release her from her many roles as spouse, mother, and professional woman.

Jesse's mother had died of cancer when Jesse was 5, leaving an older sister, two younger brothers, and a needy alcoholic father. Soon a critical, perfectionistic stepmother was added to the family. Growing up, Jesse had few of her dependency needs met. She was never allowed to grieve for her mother, nor did she recall ever being cuddled or comforted by anyone after her mother's death.

Jesse reported that in recent months she had begun to feel intense resentment in her once satisfying, long-term marriage. In her interactions with her husband and children, as well as with many of her other relationships, Jesse said she functioned as the tireless "all-giver." From an early age, she had been able to sense others' needs, and, with considerable skill, had met these needs. Now, by mid-life, Jesse felt drained and empty.

In the initial session Jesse openly expressed her despair, including her desperate need to carve out time and space just for herself. She felt that she was losing herself and was frightened. Because of the urgency of the situation I stepped in quickly with a homework assignment. I suggested that she convert an unused second floor bedroom into an art studio, complete with a sign that read "Do not enter unless I say so!" It was hoped that in this way she could begin to meet her needs in a creative way. I believed that if she could claim a safe personal space for her easel, paints, and favorite music, the need to run away in order to find herself would diminish.

Over the first 2 months, Jesse became increasingly aware of her anger at her husband, children, and all others who seemed to demand so much. In response to these feelings I encouraged Jesse to create a number of movement sequences to symbolize making space for herself in her life. Jesse felt most engaged when she did movements that portrayed pushing things away from her. Such movements gave her the feeling that she could "get some breathing room" by exerting her own will and, in this way, gain control over her own life and space. After exploring this theme through a variety of "pushing away" sequences, Jesse began to translate her movements into actual changes in her life. For example, she began to take better care of herself and started a series of expressive pastel drawings that reflected her feelings. As part of her treatment, Jesse was encouraged to make use of her natural idiom of expression, the visual arts.

The Scraping Dance. One day Jesse arrived at her session enraged. She had come to believe that she carried some sort of "psychic contamination." She said she urgently needed to scrape herself clean. Face to face with the mirroring therapist, Jesse started by scraping at her shoulders, arms, and hands, then moved to scrape her hips, pelvis, legs, and feet. She seemed to be slowly removing a thick layer of mud. After repeating this, head to toe, several times, Jesse envisioned a shower and allowed herself to relax and be rinsed by it. Her posture gradually shifted to one of openness and receiving, with palms held up and out, face lifted and smiling, and spine arched slightly backward. She ended the session by creating an imaginary cage in which she put "all those needy people." Then she joyously flaunted herself in front of the cage and, as she skipped back and forth, toward and away, she chanted, in a child's tone, "Nyah nyah, nyah nyah nyah! You can't make me feel your feelings! Those bad feelings are yours, NOT MINE."

For years, Jesse had had negative feelings about herself. In the scraping dance, she began to identify where the feelings came from and symbolically started to throw them off. But with this shift in awareness of herself new difficulties and struggles emerged.

In the next several months, Jesse was plagued by frightening images. She was not sure if the images were fantasies or partial fragments of forgotten reality. As her distress continued to escalate she reported several incidents of feeling that she was about to "fly apart," and feared that she might one day cease to exist.

In an attempt to lessen Jesse's panic I suggested an art project to be done at home. I asked Jesse to construct a series of masks representing her feelings, including the rage and sadness she had been talking about in therapy. The goal was to help Jesse distance herself from the overwhelming intensity of her emotions. I believed that by focusing her emotions on a visual art medium, a medium in which she felt comfortable, and over which she had control, she would be helped to express herself without "flying apart."

The Dark Lady Dance. A few weeks after the assignment, Jesse displayed her elaborate and imaginative handmade masks. I chose music that was percussive and asked Jesse to move to the rhythms. The "dark lady dance," as Jesse named it, developed without further prompting.

Using a series of slow Kabuki-like postures, Jesse assumed the characterization of the masks and performed three movement sequences. "Fire breath" was represented by strong, serpent-like movements of the upper torso and arms; "scissorhands" incorporated sharp cutting, slicing gestures directed downward; and finally, a cold turning away was labeled an "icy heart." Each movement theme flowed into the next as Jesse switched masks as needed.

Jesse repeated her dances for several weeks, in therapy sessions and at home on her own. Both the structure and predictability of rhythm and the once-removed character of masks helped to organize her expressive movements and channel her emotions. Jesse was learning to express vital, self-protective emotions, which until then had been forbidden.

To further counteract Jesse's fear of flying apart, I suggested movement exercises that lowered the body's center of gravity and helped her to use her weight and force more effectively. This was done by having Jesse push shoulder-to-shoulder against me. After the Dark Lady Dance, Jesse's frightening imagery lessened, as did her suicidal ideation.

As a child, Jesse had often been told not to feel and, as compensation, she tried to be "big" and took on the care-taking role. In order to keep her feelings a secret from her family Jesse had learned to "disappear," to become "selfless." To combat this tendency, Jesse decided that she needed to experience her own "healthy playpen." The playpen, she decided, must have sturdy tall rails so she could not fall out.

The Playpen Dance. Jesse began the dance by climbing inside the imagined playpen. At first cautiously, then with confidence, she explored over and over again, getting in and out. Working from a kneeling position Jesse explored the periphery, viscerally creating and discovering its strengths and height.

After many minutes of such exploration, Jesse said that if she ever flew apart again she wouldn't be afraid, "because I'm really elastic! I'll just reconsolidate, that's all!" From the safety of her symbolic enclosure, Jesse stretched up and out in an X shape, and like a toy doll with elastic bands for joints, Jesse found that she did indeed spring back to herself with every muscular release. This simple movement sequence seemed to delight her.

Over months of treatment, Jesse learned to solve many of her own problems using her own creativity. She also began to assume more of the leadership role in therapy, a healthy sign for a recovering co-dependent. Jesse's Playpen Dance provided her with the kind of early preverbal motor sequences that are thought to be critical in the formation of the self. It seemed that she was now free to experience herself in creative ways that had not previously been possible.

After 14 months of weekly sessions, Jesse reported that she no longer felt the overwhelming need to accommodate others at her own expense. As of this writing Jesse continues to find creative ways of meeting her own needs and allows herself to take personal time away from the rigors of her role as wife, mother, and professional. She reports that she has discovered her "quintessential essence."

Conclusions

Recovery from co-dependency can be a lifelong process. It begins with the discovery of the individual's true feelings and requires a continual re-negotiation of old and new relationships. It may also require the working through of traumatic memories and experiences.

Psychodramatic movement therapy lends itself to the needs of this population by eliciting and enhancing self-expression and creative capacities, by reconnecting individuals to the lost or unknown parts of themselves, and by facilitating symbolic confrontation with significant others. These elements work together to strengthen the individual's sense of self. By enabling clients to break free from old roles and helping them to constructively meet their own needs, co-dependent individuals are offered a second chance at having a life worth living.

9

Treating Anxiety: Four Case Examples

Susan Kierr

Earl Campbell drove across central Texas singing along with Willie Nelson and Waylon Jennings as their music played on his car radio. Life seemed good to the former New Orleans Saints running back. He had retired from professional football and now at age 36 he was a successful businessman. But there in his car, for no apparent reason, his heart started to race. He felt as if he were under severe stress, as if his heart was about to explode.

"I thought I was having a heart attack," Campbell later said, remembering that his father had died of a heart attack as a young man (Pope, 1991). But Earl Campbell was in good physical shape. He ran 4 miles a day, worked out, and watched his diet.

After experiencing several similar episodes, Earl Campbell started going to heart specialists. He saw four different cardiologists, and they all told him that tests showed nothing wrong. Finally, when one of the doctors recommended a psychiatrist, Campbell learned that he had an anxiety disorder.

"Anxiety" refers to an unpleasant and overriding tension that has no apparently identifiable cause. The term "anxiety disorder" is defined here as a group of illnesses that includes the type of panic disorder that Campbell had. He is among the 8.3 percent of Americans afflicted by this illness (American Psychiatric Association, 1988).

Earl Campbell is well known in the sports world because of his football fame. Since learning that he suffers from an anxiety disorder, he frequently speaks on that subject to help others identify their problem. He acknowledges that, once diagnosed, he used medication to treat his illness. This is not unusual. Physicians often prescribe tranquilizers and antidepressants to control anxiety symptoms.

Campbell's story is told to highlight another phase of his treatment. After initially receiving medications, he discovered that yoga breathing exercises gave him the control he needed, without medication. Campbell learned the effectiveness of breath work and relaxation techniques, techniques that are often part of the practice of dance movement therapy. "The thing I can't figure out is why it would happen," Campbell said in a newspaper interview. "I never dreamed I could catch anything like this" (Pope, 1991).

The "why" of anxiety disorders requires an understanding of how physiological, emotional, and cognitive factors may combine to produce the experience of anxiety. Earl Campbell is not the only one baffled by how people "catch" this disorder. Theories of causation range from biochemical imbalances to early childhood conflicts and traumas and can be divided into four categories: psychodynamic, behavioral, cognitive, and biochemical. The dance/movement therapist is trained to provide expressive activities that have an impact in all four. Relaxation techniques, body awareness, active imaging, and dramatic reenactment are some of the ways by which the anxiety disorder patient may be helped. What follows is an overview of the four theoretical areas and how each finds an avenue in treatment.

Generally, anxiety is a sense of apprehension that comes from the feeling that one's well-being is threatened. Such apprehension may be manifested in physical symptoms, including rapid heartbeat, shortness of breath, trembling, as well as irritability and nervous expectation. In addition to the panic experienced by Earl Campbell, other syndromes may be considered part of the diagnosis of "anxiety disorder." These include: phobias, posttraumatic stress disorders, and obsessive-compulsive disorders.

Panic is a sudden, overwhelming fear. Sometimes the person experiencing the panic believes he can identify a cause for the fear; at other times there is no identifiable cause. The panic usually appears when fear is experienced as a threat from which there is no escape. Victims suffer intense terror, for no apparent reason (Jarvis, 1991).

Sufferers are not able to predict when an attack will occur, though certain situations, such as driving a car, can become associated with attacks if it was in that situation that the attacks were first experienced. To protect themselves from a panic response, individuals may develop phobias. To avoid a situation that has been associated with panic, the victim restricts activities that might lead to a similar situation. For example, an experience of anxiety or panic in a crowd may cause the victim to be phobic about activities that put him/her in any busy public place. Such fear of being in crowds or public places is called agoraphobia. In an attempt to avoid public places, victims can become housebound. The four theories presented below suggest the possible origins of anxiety.

Psychodynamic Theory

Psychodynamic theory proposes that anxiety stems from unconscious conflicts related to unresolved discomfort during infancy or childhood. According to Bowlby (1963), the relationship of mother and child profoundly affects the development of the offspring's physical health, mental processes, and behavior, and, thus, the development of anxiety. Psychodynamic theory presupposes that a successful mother–child relationship is associated with the mother's ability to care effectively for her infant, emotionally as well as physically.

Though a complete discussion of psychodynamic theory is not within the scope of this chapter, it is important to understand that the psychodynamic origins of anxiety refer to the developmental or growing stages of the personality. Early unconscious or repressed unresolved conflicts appear in an adult's behavior, sometimes presenting themselves in the form of anxiety, panic, or phobia.

The psychodynamic model further suggests that a trusting and nurturing relationship between patient and therapist is significant in treatment. In this view the focus is on recreating experiences that may have been missing from the original nurturing environment. A safe and supportive place for treatment is crucial to building basic trust between therapist and patient.

As treatment progresses, this model considers the ways in which the patient's relationship with the therapist is akin to the developmental stages of the child's relationship with the parent. In therapy the patient may progress from feeling as though he or she is one with the therapist, dependent and symbiotic, to experimenting with autonomy and even leadership, separating and becoming an individual. Just as a child sometimes becomes attached to an object associated with the safety and comfort of the parent, perhaps a blanket or teddy bear, the patient may become attached to an object associated with the therapist, such as a piece of music or a drawing. These objects help to maintain the feelings of safety even when the child is away from the parent, or the patient is away from the therapist.

Behavioral Theory

Behavioral theory proposes that anxiety is a learned behavior and, as such, can be unlearned. If, for example, people are extremely uncomfortable in a particular situation or near a certain object, they learn to avoid the source of anxiety. Such avoidances may limit that person's ability to live a normal life (Ardoin, 1990). We can turn again to our example of agoraphobia. Perhaps, after an initial panic in a crowded grocery, a patient becomes afraid of crowds in other situations. He may then avoid all places where he is likely to find crowds. Staying near home becomes less anxiety-producing. The fear of crowds is thus fostered by the reinforcement of being able to reduce anxiety by staying home (Ballenger 1989).

A behavioral approach to this problem might be to picture a small crowd of people and to practice taking deep, relaxed breaths while imagining slowly moving closer to the pictured crowd. Another form of the behavioral approach is exposure therapy. In this case the patient might go near the actual feared situation, such as the crowd, while practicing the relaxation exercise. Rehearsing new behaviors and relaxation techniques while gradually increasing the size of the crowd is a form of desensitization. To practice the new behavior in front of crowds of varying sizes provides reality testing and helps extinguish the old behavior.

Cognitive Theory

Cognitive theorists study the way the brain receives, processes, evaluates, and stores information, including stressful and traumatic events. Stimulation coming into the brain may be coded both electrically and chemically, depending on the type of message. One of the cognitive functions of the brain is to organize experiences and stimuli so that they have meaning. According to Hartman and Burgess (1988), cognitive theories assume that an anxiety disorder involves an overreaction to stimuli, resulting in a thought process called "catastrophic thinking." This kind of thinking is described in life and death terms. The thoughts center on a fear that an awful, even fatal, event is going to happen. Patients frequently think, as Earl Campbell did, that something is terribly wrong with them. It is not unusual for them to fear that they are dying of a heart attack.

In cognitive theory, an intervention used to disrupt the dysfunctional response is similar to directing an inner movie in the mind, a special way of using the imagination. This process is called mental rehearsal, or visualization. The science of biofeedback has proven that such mental images do influence the autonomic nervous system, such as heartbeat, blood pressure, and brain wave patterns (Hartman & Burgess, 1988). We begin to see an overlap in cognitive theory and physiology.

It is interesting to note that the first effective treatment programs for anxiety disorders were "cognitive restructuring" techniques (Beck, 1985). This approach focuses on catastrophic thinking. When patients think something terrible is happening, they are taught to change the thought process, to restructure the way the mind is working. Cognitive therapists look at how the state of mind affects physical health. In particular, an optimistic (versus a pessimistic) way of viewing events is believed to influence the way the body responds on a biochemical level. This mind/body loop is of paramount importance in the dance/movement therapist's treatment of anxiety disorder.

Biochemical Theory

Biochemical theory suggests the presence of an underlying neurochemical dysfunction in anxiety disorders. Such a dysfunction may be the cause of the illness. For example, people with this disorder may have a "hypersensitivity" in the locus coeruleus, the part of the brain that alerts them to fearful situations and dangers. The locus coeruleus is a small sector deep in the brain that turns on and off the body's alarm system. It triggers the release of adrenaline, which steps up heart and breathing rates to provide quick energy in times of emergency. It can affect the bowels and can create dizziness, gastrointestinal symptoms, and rapid heartbeat (Ballenger, 1989).

Body chemistry, however, is affected by mental images, as noted above, and also by physical activity. For example, moving to music for 15 to 20 minutes can create a burst of adrenaline, temporarily altering the body chemistry. A "high" feeling of well-being is the result of the endorphins released in the blood stream, the brain, and the spinal fluid. This effect is increased when the movement includes having the arms lifted above the level of the heart, which raises the cardiovascular output. Aerobic dancing releases physical tension and may positively influence the mind by temporarily freeing the individual from anxiety.

Treating Anxiety

When asking the cause of anxiety disorders, the answer may not be "either/or." The operant conjunction may be "and." A person with a biological susceptibility to anxiety disorders may encounter events in childhood that then lead to particular fears. Over time these early fears may reinforce behaviors that develop into an anxiety disorder. In other words, physical and environmental conditions may combine to create an anxiety-related illness.

All four theories contribute to an understanding of anxiety and treatment can have an impact on all four areas. Sometimes a simple exercise or intervention may provide a way for the patient to work on all four aspects of functioning at once. Starting on the cognitive level, the therapist might ask a patient to visualize a peaceful landscape and then ask the person to describe details of the picture. What time of day is it? What season of the year? What are the colors, sounds, smells? Such questions, which may serve to deepen the visualization and its effect on the patient, can in turn generate a physical response. For example, if the patient imagines lying on a warm sandy beach, the muscles of the body may relax, as if on the supportive sand. The breathing rate may slow, as if following the rhythm of the waves.

Thus, a cognitive exercise that starts in the mind may proceed to affect the body, and this, in turn, may draw on elements of the person's childhood. Had there been early summers at the beach? Was there a reliable parent nearby, or was such a secure presence painfully missed? The image of the sandy beach may evoke feelings of safety now reinforced by the presence of the therapist.

Case Studies

The following cases are intended to illustrate how anxiety disorders vary and how movement interventions can apply to the various manifestations. In addition to anxiety, several of the patients cited suffered from depression and addiction; however, the primary focus of this chapter is on treating the anxiety disorder.

All the participants were either inpatients or outpatients in a psychiatric hospital, one floor of which is specifically for people with anxiety and depression. The treatment program includes traditional verbal therapy and expressive nonverbal therapies. Art, music, and dance are used to give patients a time and place to express feelings for which they may not yet have words.

Terry

Terry was 36 and lived at home with her family. Although 2 years before she had bought a house a few blocks from her parents, her new house stayed empty. She was too anxious to move out of her family's home.

An office job kept Terry busy, but she had no social life. She was frequently ill and her physician concluded that most of her physical problems, including apparent anorexia, were caused by anxiety. He recommended psychiatric care and she entered the outpatient treatment program.

Terry's days at the hospital were scheduled to begin with dance/movement therapy. She was often late and the dance studio door was closed when she arrived. When this happened, Terry stood outside the door, unable to enter. Near tears and practically motionless, Terry showed her fear in her expressive eyes and tense shoulders. Staff members learned to look for Terry in the hall. Even though she belonged inside and was expected, she was unable to knock or open the door of the room. The fact that others were in the room ahead of her seemed to stir in Terry an old need that she could not satisfy, the need to do everything perfectly and to please others.

Terry was caught in a bind: she was neither inside the room nor willing to assert herself in order to enter, much in the same way that she had her own home but could not live in it. Afraid to be late and afraid to be interruptive, she did not act to solve her problem. Her need to be "perfect" showed in other ways. Dressed with considerable care and attention to detail, Terry expressed worry about her weight and never felt thin enough. In movement sessions she was afraid to lead the group with a step or gesture of her own in case it wasn't "right." Although she seemed to long for the approval of others, Terry did not ask for it.

One morning I suggested that Terry use part of the session for a movement exercise about lateness. She hesitated, but when the group members encouraged her, she agreed to participate. The others were asked to stand in two rows to create a "lateness aisle." Terry walked down the aisle while the people forming it chanted, "You're late, you're late, you're late." As Terry walked between the two rows she looked from side to side unable to speak, her shoulders raised tensely, almost to her ears. Her arms hung stiffly and she moved with small hesitant steps.

Terry then took a place in one of the rows and the others took turns going down the "aisle of lateness." One person walked with flippant self-assuredness. Another boasted as he strolled through the aisle, describing how he had cut through traffic to get into town. One woman silently moved with long steps, arms swinging, weight leaning forward, fists clinched.

Next, I asked the group members to try one another's movement styles. Terry imitated the style that did not require words, only a bigger stride, swinging arms, and tight fists. When I suggested that each person copy the style that seemed most unlike his or her own, Terry moved between the rows shouting, "Leave me alone." Everyone applauded.

As illustrated above, role playing and dramatic techniques can be used to practice new behavior and experiment with unfamiliar situations and roles (Levy, 1979, 1988). Fear of being late had become a crippling anxiety in Terry's daily life and seemed to reflect her distress about leaving home and her fear that she was not "good" enough. She had become trapped in a cycle of anxiety, lateness, and feelings of helplessness. I chose to address the lateness anxiety because it was affecting Terry in the present.

In this exercise, Terry had a chance to practice new behaviors in a safe environment. When she experimented with more assertive ways of walking, she paved the way to be more assertive in her life. The goal of treatment was to build new responses that would be useful to her in her life outside the hospital.

Jim

Major depression occurs for more than half the patients diagnosed with anxiety disorder. It is easy to understand that symptoms of anxiety, such as panic, compulsion, and phobia, are in themselves frustrating and depressing. The disabling effect of such symptoms restricts day-to-day living, generating the helpless and hopeless feelings of depression. A biological link between anxiety disorder and depression is suggested by evidence that the same medications sometimes help both conditions (Brier, Charney, & Heninger, 1984). Likewise, people who are alcohol and drug abusers may be self-medicating.

Behaviors that suggest an individual may be suffering from anxiety, even though there is no such diagnosis, are called vulnerability markers; for example, eating disorders and alcohol and drug use. The following case shows how such markers can alert the treatment team and also demonstrates a behavioral method of binding anxiety through activity.

A tall, thin, sad man, about 50 years old, Jim originally entered the hospital on the chemical dependency unit. After going through the detoxification program, although his system tested clean of drugs and alcohol, his appearance and behavior became progressively worse. He was transferred to the anxiety and depression unit because the treatment team suspected that Jim's use of alcohol and drugs had served to give temporary relief from intense anxiety. Now he needed to work on this underlying problem.

When Jim entered the unit, he was put on medication and was expected to attend all group therapy sessions. He came to the dance studio without being asked, even stopping to remind others that it was time to start. But once in the studio he said very little and shrugged his shoulders when I asked what kind of music he liked. He stood in the circle with the others only briefly, shuffling his feet, then restlessly walked to and from the window.

At the second session Jim began looking through the cassette tapes on my desk, reading titles and artists. At the next session he began putting tapes in the player and his selections were not random. He had listened to the other patients talk about their music preferences and chose cassettes that various members of the group especially liked. He also understood when it was time for a cool-down, and he appropriately changed the tape to relaxation music. Eventually Jim knew everyone's favorites; he became the group's "disk jockey."

The therapy sessions always ended with a closing ritual. Through this repeatable and predictable movement, we marked the end of the group in a process that brought the participants together. In Jim's group the closing was usually a version of standing in a circle, holding hands, and stretching back as far as arms would permit. Patients were able to trust the hold they had on one another's hands; eyes met, breathing synchronized, and the moment of closing was acknowledged.

Although Jim was never able to move with us in the closing ritual, he created an alternative that connected him to the group. As the other patients started to make the closing circle, Jim began to put the tapes away. He timed the task precisely to end as the group finished their stretch.

As Jim's depression lifted and his anxiety decreased, his doctor continued medication, now convinced that Jim's earlier use of alcohol and drugs had been his way of treating a chemical imbalance. Jim kept his role as "dee-jay" and found other ways to help on the unit. He became an organizing force at community meetings and helped plan weekend activities. His anxiety returned only when the staff began to discuss discharge. Jim found a way to solve that problem: he became a hospital volunteer. Though he worked on a different unit, Jim continued to use his new role of group helper.

Jim was able to find a way to bind his anxiety while remaining involved with the group. He invented the role himself, reminding us that there can be no preconceived format for constructive group involvement. An activity that puts an individual in control of anxiety-producing situations may provide the anchor he/she needs in order to function. Therapy sessions create a laboratory of activities wherein the patient has a safe place to try new ways of moving and being and behaving, with no judgments and no expectations.

Adele

Adele was a frail, timid woman of 68. She was hospitalized when her anxiety reached levels that affected her marriage. Her husband had recently retired and Adele was too anxious to go places with him, even on their favorite outings. The couple became housebound. Her extreme inactivity had left Adele physically weak as well as emotionally withdrawn. The origins of Adele's anxiety were not known, but that did not mean that treatment was not available.

When Adele first talked about her anxiety, she told me that she and her husband had enjoyed going to restaurants, but for the past year, she had felt "too nervous" to go. I decided to use our individual sessions to help Adele make small steps in venturing out. I quickly discovered that Adele had a unique ability to visualize. The goal was to find positive images and their corresponding movements that would enable Adele to move beyond the safety of her hospital room.

Together Adele and I began taking short walks down the hospital corridor, in order to increase her level of activity and to regain agility in her gait, which was slow and hesitant. The cognitive task was to imagine attractive, pleasant scenes that might await her at the end of the hall.

Although I did not suggest that Adele change her style of walking, an interesting thing happened: Adele's gait acquired a new fluidity, her arms relaxed, and she started to gesture as she spoke. The relaxation in Adele's movements occurred whenever her mind was focused on images that were experienced as positive and reassuring.

At other times, when Adele was anxious, she walked the hospital hallway as if it were a dangerous place, her arms wrapped around her waist, her chest collapsed, her back curved forward, her eyes focused on the carpet as if searching for land mines. It was clear that her imagination affected her breathing, her posture, and her gait.

Because Adele seemed to walk in accordance with the pictures in her head, we worked together to change her mental images. Adele's first successful walks were those in which she visualized a park at the end of the hall, with a baby deer and its mother standing among trees. Such positive images that represented this relationship between two figures became an important part of Adele's therapy. Perhaps she saw the two deer as nurturing and harmonious because she sought that kind of relationship for herself.

One day, when Adele suggested there might be an airplane at the other end of the hall, I asked, "Where's the plane going to take you?" "To visit my grandchildren," Adele said. But as she spoke, a timidity returned to her voice and her steps got smaller. "What's happening?" I questioned softly. "It's the noise, and the airplane is so big," Adele answered. "What's scaring you?" I asked. "Getting on that airplane alone," she mumbled. When we turned around and headed back through the hallway, Adele visualized one of her favorite restaurants and the smiling maitre d' who greeted her there. The door that Adele chose as the entrance to the restaurant held symbolic meaning. It was the office of the unit social worker who was in closest contact with Adele's husband. In this way Adele counteracted her anxiety about being alone by connecting, through imagery, to her husband.

Adele practiced walking into the "restaurant," picturing her husband with her. She imagined the candlelight and heard soft music, she recalled the colors of the walls and carpet, the aromas of rich Italian cuisine, and she described the dress she would like to be wearing. Her humor returned; she reported that the head waiter was flirting with her.

Adele's hospitalization was brief. She went home with follow-up couple's sessions planned with the social worker. Adele's natural tendency to externalize her thoughts through body movement enabled her to use the visualization techniques effectively. Her treatment had an effect in both cognitive and behavioral areas, and mind and body were encouraged to work together in more positive ways.

Gina

When Gina was 27, her husband insisted on a divorce, after which she became increasingly anxious. During her three-year marriage, Gina and her husband were seldom alone, spending most of their weekends with friends, and in bars. Gina's husband liked to drink; she liked to dance. As the connection between the couple disintegrated, she criticized his drinking and he avoided her dancing. After the divorce, unable to proceed with her life, education, work, or friends, she was hospitalized for depression and anxiety.

When she came to her first session she found herself in a circle of people choosing "dance" music. Gina seemed almost euphoric. She had always thought of herself as a good dancer until her husband's unwillingness to participate undermined her confidence. Except for her refusal to drink with him, she had avoided making decisions and choices. When I asked for her preference in music, Gina said that she liked all of it. When it was her turn to lead the circle of dancers, she copied something she had seen another person doing. Yet, without realizing it, Gina embellished the movements and in so doing she invigorated the entire group.

In later sessions, Gina began to take a leadership position in the group and whenever she did so, the activity level was high. The patients danced energetically, got breathless, and expressed exuberance, while an adrenal shift in their biochemistry also marked an internal change. They discovered that dance creates a feeling of joyousness and community. "I sweat something awful but I feel so high," Gina told me. "I think I'll take a whole mess of aerobic classes and learn to be an instructor, like you." Gina identified an activity that decreased her discomfort and gave her a sense of joy and purpose. She decided to be a dance "teacher." Her enthusiasm for movement expressed hope. She discovered a new behavior, which enabled her to control her anxiety.

I continued to incorporate popular music and vigorous movement in the sessions, along with relaxation techniques. In a memorable session, Gina had an image of a field of flowers. When given paper and crayons, she drew a single red flower, then chose a song, "Lady In Red," and moved as she felt the flower would, swaying gently. This quiet movement seemed to indicate a new ability to manage her anxiety.

Later, in other sessions, additional techniques were used for relaxation. The group used exercise mats to lie on the floor and do deep breathing. I suggested isometrics, contracting and releasing muscles, as well as massage of neck and shoulders. When it was time to conclude the session with a relaxation exercise, Gina requested massage. She arranged to be sitting next to me and also took the initiative by suggesting that the group form a circle so that everyone could give and receive a massage from the nearest person. In pursuing Gina's suggestion, I was able to help the group members deal with the issue of touch, asking if everyone had heard and was interested in Gina's idea of a massage circle.

I focused on Gina's suggestion for two reasons. First, before using massage in the group, it was important for the individuals to consent to being touched. This underlined that each person had control of his or her own body and that privacy would not be invaded. The second was to support Gina's behavior in the group and to emphasize Gina's ability to get her needs met in a healthy way.

In the following weeks, Gina located a training school for massage therapists and sent for an enrollment application. Through the nurturing relationship with her therapist, Gina seemed ready to move on. To encourage this, I gave her a copy of the relaxation music played during the group massage. The music functioned as a transitional object for Gina when she was away from the hospital. She connected it to her experience of being near the therapist and the group, and this helped her to feel strong. In addition, to improve her self-esteem and ability to be independent, I frequently gave her the leadership role during sessions. In time Gina created a positive and successful self-image as a leader, a dance teacher, and a massage therapist. She gradually internalized these good feelings and learned that she could provide for herself.

Discussion

Anxiety disorder is an illness with somatic as well as emotional symptoms that often has multiple causes. Treatment includes verbal and nonverbal forms of expression and varies to meet the needs of the individuals being treated. But the approach always tries to see each person as an integration of behavior, thought, feeling, and physiology. This synthesis is essential to our understanding of anxiety disorders.

The therapist draws on techniques that have an impact in all four areas. A session may affect one or more simultaneously. Mental images, such as Adele's restaurant scenes, can be considered cognitive interventions. Activities, such as Jim's disk-jockey tasks and Terry's walk down the aisle of lateness, are behavioral. Endorphin changes, such as those created by Gina's aerobic dancing, are biochemical. Gina's tapes and Adele's nurturing images of the mother and baby deer are psychological interventions addressing developmental needs. But actually this is an oversimplification. Although placing these techniques in categories is helpful for teaching students about the differences between cognitive, behavioral, psychodynamic, and biochemical approaches, in fact individuals are not neatly divided into separate parts.

None of the techniques used in treatment happen in isolation. All individuals are intricate combinations of their biochemistry, learned behaviors, cognitive experiences, and psychodynamics. When we affect one we are simultaneously influencing all the others. This process promotes growth and change in all areas.

10

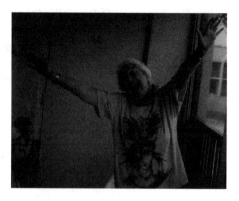

Dance/Movement Therapy with Aging Populations

Susan L. Sandel and Amy Scott Hollander

Movement is a meaningful part of many different treatment modalities for the aged. Although physical therapy, "fitness" programs, creative movement, and dance/movement therapy all use movement, each modality has its own goals.

Fitness programs offer exercises of varying levels of difficulty, depending on the stamina and overall health of the participants. The goals include increased mobility, improved circulation and breathing, relaxation, and release of tension. Emotional well-being, if it comes, is a by-product of better physical functioning. Although exercise programs take place in groups, the emphasis is on the individual's improvement.

Creative movement, which is widely used in nursing homes and senior centers, shares some of the goals that characterize fitness programs, but there are additional aims. A variety of movement activities, often accompanied by music, are designed to encourage creativity, spontaneity, body awareness, increased self-esteem, and social interaction (Herman & Renzurri, 1978).

Of all the modalities, dance/movement therapy has the broadest goals, integrating physiology, psychology, and sociology. Dance/movement therapy gives meaning to movement through the development of images, encourages emotional responses and the processing of the responses both positive and negative, and it facilitates and supports social interaction. Movement activities are not the primary goal of the group experience, but rather the tool for creating a therapeutic environment. This approach distinguishes dance/movement therapy from the other activities and offers a comprehensive treatment method for the elderly (Sandel & Johnson, 1987).

Aging Populations Differ. When we refer to dance/movement therapy with "older adults" or "elderly people" it is necessary to define the targeted population. There are several subgroups and their needs and goals are different.

Well-Elderly. Chronological age has less impact on a person's abilities than the effects of illness, disease, or trauma. A person, whether 65 or 85, if healthy, active, and alert, may benefit from a dance/movement therapy experience that offers an opportunity to maintain physical wellness while providing an arena for expressing creativity and increasing social interaction. Normal developmental tasks often become the focus of sessions: the expected milestones of aging, the birth of grandchildren or great-grandchildren, the loss of a spouse and peers, retirement, and the needed, but often painful, redirection of life's interests and energies.

Physically Challenged. Many older people have disabling or chronic conditions, arthritis, or other degenerative illnesses. Physical limitations, however, need not prevent participation in dance/movement therapy. An accepting, nonjudgmental atmosphere in which people feel free to function within the limits of their own capabilities is essential. When the focus is on the psychosocial values of the group, rather than on the activity, even the most physically challenged can have something to offer. In such an environment, activities such as making sounds, singing, telling stories, or simply touching one another are especially meaningful. For example, a woman paralyzed on one side said, "We get together to be together. Then we do as much as we can do. It's okay."

A critical factor in creating an accepting atmosphere is the language that the therapist uses in guiding the group. If the therapist says, "Everyone lift your right arm; now your left arm; now both arms," there might be people who can not do any one of these activities. Feeling unable to participate, these individuals may drop out or otherwise resist. If directions are offered as suggestions, it is less likely that people will feel excluded. The therapist might say, "Can we lift one arm? How about the other arm? If you can lift one arm, that's okay. Can anyone lift both arms? If not, lift one arm as high as you can. If you can't lift your arms, how about your fingers?" This approach makes it possible for participants to say, "No, I can't do this, but I can do..." As group norms develop, the participants themselves come up with suggestions that include individuals with physical limitations.

Implicit in a dance/movement therapy session with the physically challenged is the expectation that people will attempt to move and that movement stimulates their feelings about their bodies and their physical limitations. By creating an accepting atmosphere and not avoiding people's difficulties, the therapist models tolerant behavior that contributes to group members becoming more supportive of their peers.

Psychiatric Disorders. Significant differences exist between the elderly person who is clinically depressed due to the sudden onset of a traumatic illness or the loss of a spouse and the person with a long history of psychiatric disorders. For the depressed, the dance/movement therapy group can provide an opportunity to mobilize feelings of loss, anger, and frustration, express them through group activities, and gain support and validation by sharing the feelings with others.

People with chronic psychological problems, on the other hand, benefit from a dance/movement therapy program that emphasizes a consistent, orienting environment. These patients are often on antipsychotic or antidepressant medications and the medication, combined with the structured interpersonal milieu, helps such patients maintain adaptive functioning and prevents further social withdrawal and regression. Traditionally dance/movement therapy has proven to be effective for long-term psychiatric patients. It affords opportunities for simultaneous rhythmic movement, channeled expressions of emotions, and promotes socialization (Chaiklin & Schmais, 1979; Samuels, 1973).

Cognitively Impaired. People who suffer from memory loss, confusion, and other organic impairments, including Alzheimer's disease, benefit from dance/movement therapy that emphasizes consistency and predictability in time, place, leadership, and activities. Reality-orientation techniques are incorporated into sessions, especially into opening and closing rituals. For example, beginning the group with a structured interaction, such as passing around a foam ball while participants say their names, is reassuring and serves to enhance orientation.

When participating in movements that recall past mastery experiences, confused people appear more alert. Reminiscing stimulates cognitive reorganization, even if only while the person is participating in the group. Physical actions that evoke images of concrete activities such as rowing a boat, washing clothes, or kneading dough can reawaken memories of the past and provide an excellent vehicle for discussion and sharing.

For example, in one group we began a rowing motion, moving our shoulders up and down, forward and back, in a circular fashion. We gripped our hands into fists and proceeded to "row." As we moved and talked, one of the participants began to sing, "Row, Row, Row Your Boat." The others all joined in. This became a ritual in the group. Those who found the movement difficult sang...others moved without singing and others could do both; all were included.

Direct physical contact also has a dramatic organizing effect on people who drift in and out of reality. Sometimes people who appear disoriented can carry on a conversation when holding hands with another. Movement experiences involving physical contact (holding hands and swaying, patting shoulders) are often effective in engaging even the most cognitively impaired.

Frail Elderly. This term is applied to older people who have physical or mental conditions that place them at risk if unaided or unsupervised for at least part of their day. Dance/movement therapy sessions that utilize gentle movements, music, props, with an emphasis on socialization, are most appropriate for this group (Needler & Baer, 1982). The therapist avoids any direct manipulation of people's limbs, as they may be fragile, and some people require assistance in ambulation or other tasks. Even though dance/movement therapy sessions may not be physically rigorous, any at-risk elderly population should have medical clearance to participate.

Dance/Movement Therapy Techniques

The following specific techniques have proven most useful in this author's dance/movement therapy work with the elderly.

Circle Formation. A circle formation, the primary spatial structure for unison action, contributes to the feeling of group unity and increases the opportunity for eye contact. Because everyone is visible even those with hearing difficulties are able to participate by following others. People with visual impairments may be seated next to the therapist or someone in the group who can describe the activity to them. Although ambulatory participants may move into other spatial formations such as lines and spirals, or scatter around the room, the circle is desirable for beginning and ending groups. It is particularly important for physically disabled and disoriented people as it facilitates touch and communication.

Music. Music that taps into the natural inclination to respond to rhythm provides a useful stimulus for beginning a session. In fact, music with a clear rhythmic beat is the most consistently useful kind for dance/movement therapy. This should include music from the patients' pasts as well as more current music.

Vocalization. Whenever possible, participants should make sounds while moving, as even a "hum" or an "ah" stimulates breathing, circulation, and central body involvement. Any sound that a person offers can be incorporated in the group experience. As people become more comfortable with vocalization, the therapist can encourage sounds that are expressive of particular feelings. "What kind of sounds do we make when we're happy? Sad? Angry?" In combination with movements, the sounds can increase the range of expression and communication.

A vocal ritual is routinely used to end a movement group that takes place in a day-treatment program. We raise our arms to the ceiling as our voices get louder and louder. As our arms come down our voices get softer and softer. Often participants forget the softer and softer but give out a good strong yell. Larry, a man with advanced Alzheimer's disease, is particularly loud. He holds the yell for a good 30 seconds, and ends with a smile on his face, feeling his power. Most participants love to yell and end the group smiling and laughing.

Props. Certain props are particularly useful for stimulating activity and encouraging interaction among the elderly. Some favorites are foam "Nerf"™ balls, colored scarves, and various lengths of stretch material (Caplow-Lindner, Harpaz, & Samberg, 1979). These objects may be used to motivate movements such as squeezing, punching, tugging, and throwing, and to develop participatory games. Any of the props may provide increased sensory stimulation and serve to link group members together to increase interpersonal awareness.

In groups with disoriented or confused patients, props may be the external focus or support that keeps the group together. In sessions with more alert people, props may serve as the initial stimuli for interaction but may not be necessary later on as group members begin to interact freely with one another.

Empathic Movement. One of the major characteristics that distinguishes dance/movement therapy from other body disciplines is the therapist's reliance on empathic movement as the basis for group interaction. Developed by pioneer dance therapist Marian Chace, empathic movement is a technique in which the therapist guides and develops group interaction as it unfolds during the session. Therapists do not come to a session with a preconceived plan of activities but rely on verbal and nonverbal cues from the participants for the contents of the session. Suggestions, rather than commands, characterize this approach, so that the therapist serves as catalyst, not teacher.

The therapist first creates an atmosphere that encourages self-expression through movement. Then the therapist responds to the feelings and thoughts being expressed, but does not impose specific muscle movements to condition postural changes or evoke certain emotions. This technique challenges the therapist's skills in dealing with both spontaneous movement expressions and group process (Sandel, 1993a).

Imagery. The development of group images is another distinguishing technique of dance/movement therapy. The use of imagery shifts the experience from simple action to a symbolic, shared act. A basic guideline for this technique is to begin with the movement and allow the image to develop out of the action. For example, if the group movement involves stamping feet, the therapist might ask, "What can we stamp on?" or "Have you ever stamped on something?" The questions encourage participants to express ideas and associations without binding the group to the therapist's imagination. Imagery is also useful in identifying feelings, relating movements to real situations, and facilitating reminiscence. Thus, the development of images gives significant meaning to the movements (Sandel, 1993b). For example, in a group with confused participants, the therapist danced with a woman in the center of the circle. As they danced, they talked playfully about what they would wear to the "ball." The woman, who had dementia and rarely recounted events from her past, described in detail a blue satin gown she had once worn.

Reminiscing. As in the example above, dance/movement therapy provides an opportunity for reminiscing in a social context. Reminiscing can be an adaptive behavior and should be encouraged (Butler, 1963; Fallot, 1976; McMahon & Rhudick, 1967). Reminiscing also aids in developing interaction among the participants. For example, rhythmic actions done in unison uncover forgotten memories and feelings, memories that may be pleasant or painful or of past experiences of mastery.

The principal that applies to imagery applies here: Always begin with the movement and allow the reminiscence to develop from the action. Progression from the sensory experience of movement to the symbolic image or association emerges from the spontaneous unfolding of material. For example, in a group of frail elderly who were seated in chairs, marching in place elicited a tremendous response. To the music of "Here we go, into the wild blue yonder..." foot stomping intensified. Ralph, who could not walk due to a stroke, stamped his feet rhythmically. Gertrude moved her feet despite a fractured hip. The energy level increased in the room and everyone "marched."

Case Examples

The following is taken from a therapy session with five women, ages 78 to 92, all nursing-home residents. Four of the five were confused, and three had diagnoses of organic brain syndrome. All of the women experienced extensive periods of disorientation, and several did not know where they were until they entered the therapy room. Three of them participated minimally in verbal conversations, whereas one had lengthy spells of total muteness. All had been attending the movement-therapy group weekly for at least 6 months.

We began by lifting our arms up and down slowly as part of our warm-up. I added a suggestion that we raise our arms as if we were lifting something very heavy and then proposed that we pass the heavy object around the circle from one person to the next. When I asked, "What can we pass?" Ms. D. said, "A sack of potatoes." As we continued, Ms. D., who had grown up on a farm in Ireland, told the group about potato farming. She described the process of planting, digging, and storing the potatoes in the barn covered with hay. When she finished I asked the group, "What else can we do with the potatoes?" Ms. S. started throwing imaginary potatoes across the circle, an action that was picked up by the rest of the group and caused much laughter, even from Ms. K., who had been mute.

When I asked if we could do anything else with the potatoes, someone suggested mashing, and everyone proceeded to "mash" the potatoes, with several offering ingredients such as butter and salt, and giving directions concerning proper preparation! When I asked what we could do next, Ms. S. said gleeful-ly, "Eat them!" and the women began "feeding" the mashed potatoes to one another.

Discussion followed:

Ms. K: I'm a good cook. I can make soup.

Ms. S: I used to like to cook.

Therapist: Did anyone else like to cook?

Ms. C: I was a good cook once.

Ms. S: (Turning to Ms. C., her roommate) M., you never told me you cook! (She looked respectfully at Ms. C.)

Ms. D: I did a lot of cooking. You know I have nine children. I used to like to feed them spinach in the winter; it was good for them.

Therapist: What else did you feed them?

Ms. D: I baked pies. Apple pies, with potato in the crust.

The conversation then shifted to a current concern—the food in the nursing home.

Ms. S: They gave us apples today—apples in a dish. It's not real apple pie (she paused, looked around, and made a face). I ate it anyway! (Big smile.)

The group responded with giggles and nods.

Of significance is that these five women, supported by the structure of the movements and periodic interventions by the therapist, were able to sustain a logical sequence of cognitive and motor activity that lasted for 20 minutes. Even the less verbal people contributed to a conversation organized around the memory of past competencies. Ms. S.'s regard for her roommate clearly increased when she learned that Ms. C. had been a good cook. Repeatedly, in such situations, residents learn about each other's accomplishments for the first time. The resulting interaction can be a first step toward socialization for peo-ple who have been socially isolated (Sandel, 1978).

Reminiscing, of course, is not always linked to positive experiences; it can also evoke painful memories. In many institutions there are few opportunities for aged residents to express negative affect in a constructive way. Because angry outbursts and abusive language are abhorred by most residents and staff alike, many patients fear that they would be viewed as "impolite" or "ungrate-ful" if they openly expressed negative feelings or critical attitudes. The intima-cy that evolves in small groups through sharing memories creates an atmos-phere in which upsetting feelings and complaints may be aired.

In a more alert group of seven residents, male and female, who ranged in age from 77 to 95, the first expression of negative affect occurred after the group had been meeting weekly for many months. The following took place during the 14th month.

Each person took turns leading warm-up exercises, which included a variety of movements such as talking to others with our hands. While we did this, there was talk of the many residents who had the flu. The talk developed into symbolic action of throwing and pushing the sickness away from the members of the group.

Mr. J: Push it away; pull it back.
Mr. L: Why the hell do you want to pull it back?
Mr. J: Okay, push it away and leave it there!

I suggested that we extend the movement so that we were rocking forward and back in our chairs. One woman mentioned that it was an awful feeling to fall, and recounted an incident in which she had fallen badly. I asked if anyone else remembered a fall. Mr. J. remembered going iceskating and falling backward on the ice. Ms. K. and Mr. L. both shared their memories of breaking an arm in a fall.

Ms. B: I don't remember falling. I was always very careful.
Mr. J: (In a joking tone) You're a fallen woman!
Ms. B: I should hope not (laughing). That would be something, wouldn't it!
(Everyone laughed, conversed, with neighbors.)

What is important here is not only the specific content of what was discussed, but also the fact that people were able to share unpleasant memories while maintaining a sense of humor in a spontaneous and largely unselfconscious manner. The reminiscences developed from the sensorimotor experiences and provided a focus around which the interaction occurred.

In another group of confused patients, we were exercising our legs by lifting one foot after the other.

Mr. H: This reminds me of marching.
Ms. G: Aren't we too old to march anymore?
Ms. F: No.
Therapist: Did anyone ever march in a parade or a procession?
Mr. H: In the army. (He sings. "When the Caissons Go Marching Along," and several people join him.)
Therapist: (The group continued stamping their feet.) Anyone else ever march in a procession?

Ms. M: I know I have, but I can't remember. Maybe in school, yes school.
Therapist: Perhaps in a graduation procession?
Ms. M: Yes, that's it.
Ms. V: There were processions in Italy when Hitler came to power. All the soldiers marched down the streets. And processions for Mussolini.
Therapist: Can we march like soldiers? (The group responded with louder, more militant stamping.)
Ms. V: And then there were processions in Israel for the Jews who were killed by Hitler. (She started to cry.) Many of my people were killed there, in Europe.
(A co-therapist and patient on either side of her extended their hands to her, as the rest of the group stopped stamping.)
Co-therapist: It's understandable that you feel sad about that.
Ms. V: I'm sorry to trouble you with my problems. They say I talk too much.
Co-therapist: Who says that?
Ms. V: They all do.
Ms. S: We like hearing your stories.
Therapist: It's okay to tell us.
Ms. V: Thank you.

Although the reminiscence was not fully explored at that time, the value that painful memories can be shared and that group members are willing to listen was supported by the group. Despite the impact of Ms. V.'s associations, the group did not fall apart, and Ms. V. seemed much relieved when her pain was openly acknowledged (Sandel, 1978).

The reminiscing that develops from movement also leads to discussion about current issues in the participant's lives. The activity itself and the memories it stimulates can be used by the therapist to facilitate here-and-now interactions.

Joe, a 79-year-old man with a primary diagnosis of Alzheimer's disease, began attending a dance/movement therapy group in a specialized day program. He was tall and slim and, despite his dementia, was physically fit. He had owned a company and had been clever and well-liked by his employees. Because Joe was deaf in one ear he had difficulty following oral instructions but followed the movements when he could see the therapist. When he moved he often smiled and sometimes sang or told a story. Over and over he told about "during the war" when he was involved in intrigue and was sometimes in danger. (The information was confirmed by his family.) Joe's story of his exciting past stimulated the admiration of others. As his self-confidence was bolstered by their admiration, Joe began to get up on his feet and dance with the therapist and with any able group members. He began to initiate movements and exert leadership. Others respected him and asked his opinion about things that concerned them.

Although Joe declined physically over the next 4 years, he continued participating in the daily group. The structure and routine, as well as his role in the group, helped him to maintain his self-esteem. A few months ago, Joe suffered a stroke that partially paralyzed his left side. With encouragement from the group, he used his right arm to raise his left arm and assist in lifting his left foot. This effort contributed to his rehabilitation and further enhanced the admiration and respect of his peers.

Conclusions

All elderly people, even those limited by physical, cognitive, or mental disabilities, can function in a dance/movement therapy session. The human response to rhythm, music, and touch is enduring and transcends the effects of aging.

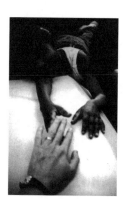

Part 2

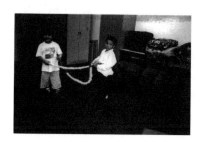

Children

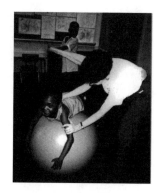

11

Sue and Jon: Working with Blind Children

Judith Pines Fried

Imagine for a moment that you live in darkness, that you were born in darkness. How would your world seem to you? How would you know where you are in relation to people, to objects? How did you, as a baby, learn to know and love your mother? How did you express love and attachment? How did you receive and send messages to others? How did you learn that something that existed yesterday still exists today? Without the sense of sight we rely on our other familiarly known senses: hearing, touch, taste, and smell, and we have a less widely recognized sense—the sense of movement.

Until the 1960s, there had been no in-depth, comprehensive studies of the infant blind to equal those begun by Professor Selma Fraiberg and her colleagues (Adelson & Fraiberg, 1974, 1976; Fraiberg, 1968, 1976, 1977; Fraiberg & Freedman, 1964; Fraiberg, Siegel, & Gibson, 1966: Fraiberg, Smith, & Adelson, 1969). Fraiberg's careful developmental approach offers answers to many of the questions posed above and the insights made available by her studies have implications beyond the specific population: infants otherwise intact but blind from birth. Fraiberg's findings can be of special value to the therapist working with this and other populations.

Infants Born Blind:
Some Concepts of Development

The developmental tasks of the blind infant are the same as those of the sighted infant. For both, ego refers to the self, especially as distinct from the world and from other selves. And ego may be further defined as that division of the psyche that is conscious and most in touch with reality. Ego formation refers to the process by which the newborn, through sensory and environmental experiences, gradually develops those structures that tell us who and where we are in the world.

According to Freud (1932,1964), the earliest task of the ego is "to observe the external world [and] lay down an accurate picture of it in the memory traces of its perceptions" (p. 75). The central figure in this "external" world is, of course, the mother. The blind infant may "lay down an accurate picture" of the mother, but this picture can in no way resemble the picture made by the sighted child. What might the difference between the visual and the nonvisual picture mean for the mother/child relationship? And what does it mean for the developing ego? When speculating on the earliest life experiences of the child who is born blind, then, the question arises: Can the developing ego find its way in total darkness? Can the sighted mother be expected to light the way?

Fraiberg (1977) writes that in an ordinary mother/child relationship, the dialogue between them depends on the visual signals that are exchanged. The nursing infant learns to know the mother's face, beaming and attentive. The mother, in turn, is rewarded by the sight of her infant's first smiles. Fraiberg asks:

> When the signals are obliterated through the blindness of the baby, what happens to the discourse between the child and the mother?...In what ways might blindness become an impediment to the development of human attachments? And if the pathways to human attachment are not found...the essential conditions for ego formation will be lacking. (1977, p. 70)

In other words, all of the natural forms of mother/child communication that evolve for the normal child are at risk for the child born blind.

Developmental Milestones

In the early 1960s, Fraiberg and her fellow researchers found evidence that forever changed earlier explanations of two important developmental hallmarks: smiling and stranger anxiety. It had been generally believed that an infant's earliest smiles are elicited by the sight of a human face (Spitz, 1965), and that it is the baby's later ability to distinguish between a familiar and an unfamiliar face that is demonstrated by the infant's discomfort, called stranger-anxiety. Fraiberg (1977) states that at 6 to 8 weeks the blind baby lights up at the sound of his mother's voice and clearly prefers it to all other voices. The smile occurs, according to Fraiberg, if the mother talks to and cuddles her baby enough so that the baby can "know" her. By 8 months, this same infant demonstrates all the classic signs of stranger anxiety when the voice of anyone who is not the mother or father is heard.

The blind infant also pulls up to and lets down from a standing position, and shows a readiness-to-creep posture, all on schedule and without special assistance. Other developmental sequences do not appear on cue, however.

In the born-blind population all locomotor skills are delayed. The reason is that for all infants, sighted or blind, reaching and grasping are preliminary to locomotion. It is the object out of reach that first motivates the infant to move. Even with special assistance, the blind baby does not reach and grasp until he has lived twice as long as his sighted counterpart—10 to 12 months versus 5 to 6 months. At 5 months a sighted infant reaches for a rattle, having learned that the rattle is an object. But the blind 5 month old does not know the object is out of reach, does not even know the object exists. By 10 to 12 months, the blind baby does reach and the event is noteworthy. It is more complex to associate an object with sound than it is to make the same association through sight. Even the sighted child does not respond to an object from sound cue alone until the same age as the blind infant (Fraiberg, et al., 1966). In other words, no infant, sighted or blind, will be motivated to reach or crawl until some object out of reach is perceived as real and desirable. For the blind child, *object concept* is always delayed.

Object concept is thought of as the individual's ability to recognize some thing, be it mother or toy, as separate from the self, distinct and apart. *Object permanence* refers to the ability to know that the same object exists even when it is neither seen, heard, nor felt. A sighted baby, seeing his mother leave the room, may surprise his mother by crawling after her. But the blind baby, having no visual concept of an object—or mother—moving in space, will be still. Thus, creeping often never occurs and independent walking may be delayed until the second or third year. The results of these delays are far reaching.

Mobility and the Motor Urge

At the time when other infants are starting to creep to the toy or to the mother, the blind infant is also on all fours, but he is "rocking ready to go but with no place to go" (Fraiberg, 1977, p. 278). This may mark the onset of stereotyped rocking and other repetitive movements that are often called "blindisms." The persistence of such movements may be explained, in part, by the theories of Mittelman (1954, 1957), a researcher who looked at the motor development of both blind and sighted children. Mittelman postulates that movement, or what he terms "motility," is an urge in its own right, an urge that operates essentially in the same way as a drive or instinct. Evidence of the motor urge may be seen in the so-called random movements of infants and in the often rhythmic or circular motions of young children. Such bouncing, jumping, and turning seem to serve no visible purpose aside from the experience of the movement itself (Mittelman, 1954). Although present at all ages, the motor urge is predominant in the second and third years of life when rapid development of motor skill and mobility paves the way for the mastery of movement, reality testing, and impulse control. It may well be that the frustration of this urge also paves the way for the stereotyped, impulse-driven activities that characterize much of the born-blind population.

The inhibiting effect of blindness on mobility has another result. Visual clues provide the most common indicators of the presence or absence of the mother and of the presence or absence of danger. A toddler who feels the safety of his mother nearby will feel free to move and explore and, thus, manifest the motor urge appropriately. The blind infant, deprived of this feeling of safety, manifests the motor urge not by motility but through the continuation of vigorous repetitive mannerisms.

Fraiberg (1977) suggests a similar period of "postural readiness," the "ready to go" period referred to above. She states that she observed "motor stereotypies in the blind baby during these periods of postural readiness and no mobility" (p. 277). Fraiberg suggests that there are serious developmental hazards associated with substituting stereotyped movements for purposeful mobility. Chief among these may be the fate of aggression.

Aggressive Discharge

Fraiberg and her fellow researchers hypothesize that from the time of the infant's earliest expressions of aggression, a time when the infant goes from passively sucking to actively biting, the sighted infant begins to transfer from the mouth—as the aggressive mode of expression—to the muscular system. This transfer is facilitated by the progress in locomotion that occurs during this period: readiness to crawl followed by crawling (Adelson & Fraiberg, 1976; Fraiberg, 1968; Fraiberg & Freedman, 1964). In the blind, however, this readiness, as noted above, is followed by absence of locomotion. What, then, is the fate of a blind child's natural aggression? By the time locomotion is achieved, is it too late for normal aggressive drives to be linked to mobility so that healthy discharge can occur?

Most researchers answer these questions by suggesting that if the delay in mobility is too long, healthy discharge finds a substitute in the inappropriate discharges, the motor stereotypies so prevalent in the young blind child (Adelson & Fraiberg, 1974, 1976; Burlingham, 1961; Fraiberg, 1977). In addition to serving as substitutes for normal aggressive outlets, these stereotyped behaviors are often utilized by the blind child in other ways. They serve to ward off or shut out unpleasant stimuli, thus providing the blind child with a muscular defense system. Like any defense system, this system not only serves to protect the child from discomfort, but also isolates him from growth experiences. The lack of timely mobility contributes to two other core problems for the blind child: the development of an intact body image and the development of language.

Body Image and Language Development

Body image has been defined as "the concept which each person has of his own body as an object in space, independently and apart from all other objects" (Hinsie & Campbell, 1974, p. 379). Another definition emphasizes awareness of body parts and their relationship to one another (Hapeman, 1967); whereas another includes both aspects, defining body image as "a knowledge of body parts, how the parts relate to each other… and how the parts relate to the spatial environment" (Mills, 1970, p. 46). Other theorists stress the importance of body-image development to ego development and to the individual's ability to differentiate self and nonself (Adelson & Fraiberg, 1974, 1976; Fraiberg, 1977).

Whatever the definition, it seems evident that blindness inhibits normal body perception. Fraiberg writes:

> Body image is constructed by means of the discovery of parts and a progressive organization of these parts in coherent pictures…For the blind child there is no single sense that can take over the function of vision in replicating body image. (1977, pp. 268-69)

What then, does it mean for the blind child if an intact body image does not develop? How does this child come to know "self" and "other" so that ego formation can proceed? The sighted 2 year old discovers and is enchanted by his image in the mirror. He soon recognizes himself as an entity as distinct as that much-longer recognized entity, his mother. This dual recognition seems to be a necessary precondition if the young child is to understand what we mean by "I" and "you." The lack of such recognition may explain the blind child's frequent misuse of pronouns long past the age when the sighted child has mastered this aspect of language. A blind child's pronoun usage, then, can raise questions and provide clues as to the child's differentiation of self from others as well as to the child's body image.

As with other developmental milestones, the blind child's acquisition of language both parallels and diverges from the sighted child's, much in the same way that motor development both parallels and diverges (Burlingham, 1961; Fraiberg, 1977). Babbling and jabbering, as well as word imitation, all occur within the first year for both populations. Fraiberg points out that:

The vocal dialogue which is available to the blind baby and his parents is, finally, the one channel which remains open and available as a relatively undistorted language system between mother and child. (1977, p. 109)

After the first year, however, delays in the blind child's language occur. During the second year, when sighted children typically show a spurt in vocabulary, blind children's language begins to show the consequences of their deprived status. Burlingham (1972), reporting on her work at the Hempstead Clinic in London, writes that blind children "seem to forget the few words they have learned already or, at least, do not increase them" (p. 296). Burlingham goes on to say that this delay seems "influenced by the restriction and inhibition in motor development" (p. 296). How or why this occurs she does not speculate.

There is another noteworthy peculiarity that sometimes occurs in the blind child's language, called "echolalia" or "echolalic speech." Echolalia is unlike imitation that is normal to a year-old child. During the process of learning to talk, an infant repeats the mother's sound, trying to produce a word or name an object. Echolalia is more akin to parroting, in which the words are reproduced without seeming to have meaning.

Fraiberg (1977) suggests that the lack of vision and the delay in mobility conspire to create the delay in language that reflects the blind child's devastating "experiential poverty" (p. 222). Thus, we see that the resultant problems in the development of the ego and the concept of self add to the blind child's difficulties in communicating, in joining the world of sighted peers.

A Picture of the Blind Child

It is evident that many of the unique problems of this population are directly traceable to restrictions on mobility, to issues of body image, to coping with aggressive urges, and, finally, to poverty of communication within the most significant of all relationships—that between the infant and the mother. Born without the organizing function of vision, how does the blind child appear to the sighted world? Reporting on their extensive observations of blind children, Gruber and Moore offer the following:

> This child has communication problems. He often retreats into silence or becomes so vocal that he intrudes with noises into any environment....Where he has developed speech patterns, he may repeat what is said to him or fail to make expected use of pronouns...
>
> This child...may identify his own boundaries with self abuse. He may pinch and scratch himself until he bleeds...he may fill the empty space with repetitive motions...or flick objects close to his ears to enjoy the pleasure of sound which he can make for himself at his own will. This child, jumping not for joy, but lack of anything else to do, may curl up in quietness on the floor...so still he seems not to breathe. (1963, pp. 3–4)

The sections that follow concentrate on two anopthalmics (born without eyes), their case histories, and the therapy work done with them over a 6-month period.

Blind Children's Center

Founded in 1938, Blind Children's Center consists of an infant development program, a preschool for children to age seven, and a limited residential program. Psychotherapy is regularly available for the children, as needed. Counseling with a social worker is ongoing for all families. An internship for dance/movement therapists was available at the time I worked at the Center.

The Children

When first at the Center, I was asked to work with two seven year olds—Jon and Sue—both in the same preschool class. At the outset, by tacit understanding with the teacher, I only observed, was not introduced to the children or in any way acknowledged as being present, a situation I came to appreciate as it gave me time to watch and learn. All the children in the preschool were accustomed to visitors so my presence caused no disruption. After several days I was introduced casually and began to interact with the children in the yard, at first, and then in the classroom. It seemed a long preliminary before being permitted to start sessions with the children, but time served us well.

The following observations are based on notes made during the preliminary observation period. Sue is a highly socialized child. She talks to everyone, calls people by name, recognizes not only voices but footsteps in the hall. She is volatile and moody, loves to tease and be teased, is stubborn and whiny, and able to make her demands known. She asks the teacher for attention: "What's for lunch?" "What's that noise?" She is restless and exhibits repetitive rapid twiddle-flipping movements in arms and hands that do not carry over into her torso—the movements are gestural and bound.

Sue moves easily about the Center. She asks to go to the kitchen to find out "what's for lunch" and to the office "for a drink." Both journeys require considerable navigational skill and bring social rewards in the form of praise and affection from the kitchen and office staff.

Often noisy, Sue is given to shrieks and shouts. She can identify and imitate sounds in her environment, has a great curiosity about new sounds, and listens to all music intently. She imitates staff and other children with uncanny accuracy.

Despite her vitality and social skills, I was left with a crucial question, written in the margin of the notes: Why does she seem so sad in the midst of all this ruckus?

Jon gave a completely different picture. I wrote: He is like a cloud. Jon's "flipping" (as the teacher called all stereotyped behaviors, regardless of their form) is much different from Sue's. He pats every surface softly. He twiddles small objects near his mouth, wiggles a foot when told by his teacher to "stop flipping." He seldom calls anyone by name or even speaks voluntarily. He does not make conversation, the way Sue does. When he does speak, Jon's tone is flat and affectless with little variation in pitch, in contrast to Sue's wide tonal and affective range. There is a gentle, pliant quality to Jon; his resistance is in non-doing. He demands and receives little attention, unlike Sue. He generally does what he is told, but quietly and without enthusiasm. He will use language when directed to do so and use correct pronouns only when told. The effect is of obedient docility, without any real investment—a sort of echolalia-on-command.

As with Sue, a note in the margin: Jon looks happy in a way that Sue does not, as if in a secret world of his own. He is inside his own place, doing his own thing—pat, pat, pat.

Case Information

What follows was transcribed just after starting work with the children, from the files of Doctor M., the director of the Infant Development Program, and from information given informally by the teachers.

Sue was a full-term baby; the delivery was "easy; there was no evidence of illness or drug-taking by the mother during her pregnancy." Other than the anopthalmia, there was no observable abnormality. She had an older sister, no age given, who was normal. Sue was brought to the Center at 3 ½ months. Her development was considered "normal to date." She had smiled at her mother's voice at 8 weeks, had "head control" at 3 months. Her primary stimulation was music; her mother played rock-and-roll on the radio most of the day and night. The mother reported that "Sue lies in the crib and listens."

Sue was brought to the Center at intervals for a year, during which time she was regularly evaluated and the parents were taught techniques to assist her development. At 15 months she could "move backwards on her tummy or in a walker"; she fed herself and held her own bottle. She had a vocabulary of about half-a-dozen words, including "daddy" and her sister's name; but she did not say "mama." Doctor M. reported herself to be "very satisfied with Sue's development."

After the 15-month evaluation, no appointments were kept for 7 months, at which time the doctor wrote that she was "appalled by Sue's regression." Now, at nearly 2 years, she was biting herself until she had raw spots on her hands. She was using "much self-stimulation to shut out the environment; covered her ears and bit everyone in the family." She did not walk alone, fed herself only now and then; was not using a cup or spoon. Doctor M. was very concerned about the self-destructive behaviors and urged the parents to bring Sue to the Center weekly.

Sue did not return, however, for 5 months, at which time she was 2 years, 3 months old. Her mother reported that Sue had been sleeping with her parents "until recently" but now slept alone if the radio was on all night. She had started to walk holding on to furniture, called family members by name, was not biting but was "flipping" with her hands.

Again there was a lapse of contact and Sue was not seen again until she was 4. At that time Doctor M. persuaded the parents to enroll her in the preschool. Sue was not toilet trained, did not dress herself, and "flipped constantly" (report from teacher). She was very attached to her mother, her sister, and a grandmother. The doctor's evaluation was that Sue's delay was "mostly on an emotional basis."

When I first met Sue, 3 years had passed, she was 7 and there had been radical changes in her and in her life. She seemed the most socially developed child at the Center, interested in and able to initiate contact with all of the adults and most of the children. She toileted herself and was a tidy eater, using spoon or fork. But 2 months prior to our first meeting, Sue's mother had committed suicide, at which time her sister and her grandmother had gone to live in Texas. Sue was now spending weeknights at the Center and weekends with her alcoholic father and his girlfriend. I was not fully informed of Sue's circumstances until just before we began therapy sessions; there was ample reason for the sadness noted in earlier observations. But whatever her life situations, Sue was the kind of child who took up a lot of room at the Center. She was not a child to ignore or forget.

Jon, on the other hand, seemed undemanding to the point of having little substance. Although Sue was a child who would always be attended, Jon could easily be ignored.

Jon was born after a difficult pregnancy; his brothers, both normal, were 4 and 5 at the time of his birth. There was no family history of blindness or ill-health, and there were no postnatal complications. He was brought to the Center when he was a year old, at which time Doctor M. noted he was a "normally developing anopthalmic with some problems in the family that can be remedied with appropriate help." Jon had smiled at 2 months, turned over at 6 months; played pat-a-cake at 9; sat unsupported and pulled up at 10 months; said "dada" and "mama" at 11 months; he was cruising and working with both hands at a year—all normal for that age. However, Jon never crawled and at his first Center visit, he did not finger-feed or hold a bottle either.

To help with the family's "problems," the doctor encouraged Jon's mother to support his independence and not to overprotect him. Two months later Doctor M. reported that he was "doing well emotionally and physically." The parents gave him more freedom for exploration and "Jon seems a happy child." At 17 months there was a language spurt but Jon used the word "Baba" for all three women who cared for him, his mother, maternal grandmother, and a neighbor. At this time he cruised when hand held and he stood alone. The doctor referred to him as a "normally developing child in all areas."

Seven months later, when he was 2, the doctor was "concerned." Jon had regressed. He no longer walked and had made no progress in feeding himself. His mother resisted suggestions that he be allowed to go hungry until he did feed himself. The doctor also reported, however, that she found his cognitive development entirely adequate. Jon began preschool at this time and his teacher from that period told me that his "parents' attitude, especially his mother's, wasn't good for him." His parents, according to the teacher, believed Jon to have been "sent by God as a test of their faith." For this reason, no one in the family treated Jon in any way as a "normal child" but rather more like what the teacher characterized as a "sacred object." There were no further case notes after this time. The teacher who had worked with Jon in her group when he was 5, said he had changed little from 5 to 7, when I met him. In fact, his language had continued to slip and he engaged more and more in continuous hand motions.

The differences between Sue and Jon could not have been greater and their styles of self-stimulation seemed to perfectly match their personalities. Sue flipped her hands and arms with quick vigorous movements that did not carry over to the rest of her body, which seemed stiff and held. Jon, on the other hand, patted with light, less rapid movements that resonated throughout his body. In their histories there was one marked similarity: Both children, according to Doctor M., progressed well and then, at age 2, regressed.

The timing of both children's regressions seemed to support Fraiberg's (1977) and Mittelman's (1964) speculations regarding the onset of stereotyped behaviors. At the time of the motor urge both children were denied, by reason of their blindness, the free expression of mobility and all that it meant for their development. The other difficulties one could expect to follow had, in fact, followed. Thus armed with case notes, first-hand observations and some reading in the field, I began to work with these two 7 year olds.

The Therapy

The room allotted for therapy was upstairs at the Center in a room not ordinarily used by the children. It was a staff lounge and full of furniture that when pushed back, yielded a free, carpeted space of about 6 by 9 feet. There was a table high enough for both child and therapist to crawl under. The couch and one chair were covered in a vinyl material, which when slapped, gave off a percussive sound. The furniture and the open space all played a part in the therapy.

Sessions with Sue

By the time we went to the therapy room for the first time, Sue and I were, at least nominally, friends. When told we were "going to do movement," she asked, "What's movement?" I touched her flipping hand, saying, "That's movement." She came willingly but seemed uneasy in the unfamiliar room and refused to take off her shoes. To ease her anxiety, I began to sing and Sue moved to sit in my lap, cuddled briefly, and demanded, " Sing it again!" When the song finished, she sat up and started to flip her hand close under her chin. I tried the movement, which she seemed to hear, and she stopped. And I stopped. When she started again, I did too. She announced, "You are doing it wrong!" I said." You are better at it than I am, maybe you can teach me." We spent time then and in future sessions in this "teaching" but Sue made it clear that I was not able to master her rapid hand motion to her satisfaction. The flipping, however, provided a starting point for making a relationship with Sue on a movement level and, specifically, as a starting point from which to enlarge the movement, carrying it into other body parts and, in time, to begin to explore the space.

In that first session there were two other events that proved important for our work. Without planning to do so, I began our first session by singing to Sue. It started with our trip up the stairs, with a simple folk-type song about the activity. It seemed to help and from then on everything I said to Sue was in song.

The other event occurred near the end of the session when Sue said her mother was "at the market to buy cereal." I made no comment at the time, but after the session inquired of the teacher as to how they were dealing with the suicide. The teacher said, "Sue has the information, but may not 'know.'" In this same conversation with her teacher, we discussed Sue's unwillingness to take off her shoes. The teacher said that Sue seemed to have difficulty sometimes knowing if her shoes were part of or separate from her body. This suggested that Sue's body image was unstable.

In the next session, Sue came eagerly but still refused to take off her shoes. She asked me to sing, "Eentsy-Weentsy Spider," which I did; we held hands or touched feet as I led actions to the words of the song, changed to fit the movements. I hoped, in this way, to answer some of my questions about her body image, and, at the same time, to enlarge her movement range and ease whatever it was—tension, anger, or grief—she was holding in her body. Sitting on the floor, we played with her "flipping," making it fast and slow, large and small, near and far. Suddenly Sue said, "Sing a song" and I sang "Hush Little Baby." She listened, slumped and very still. When the song ended, she sat up and said, "I'm waiting for my mommy." "I know about your mommy," I said, to which Sue did not respond in any way. "You must miss her very much." Sue began her flipping gestures but did not otherwise seem to react. "Do you cry?" I asked. She said "Yes" and crawled into my lap. I sang "we are rocking," and we continued to rock until it was time for the session to end.

Neither of us mentioned Sue's mother in the following session, but she did take off her shoes for the first time. This could be a clue. If the issue of her shoes suggested an unstable body image, perhaps this body image was connected to a question of her mother and of safety in an unstable world. In the session after that, she asked for "Hush Little Baby," which I sang while we stood holding hands and swaying. Then she said, "Sing Sue misses mommy." From that time on, she asked for those words or elaborations thereof in nearly every session, sometimes at the start and sometimes just before it was time to go.

Although Sue was now able to take off her shoes for most, though not all, sessions, she remained reluctant to move about in the room unless she was fully on the floor, lying or crawling, or if we were holding hands. This was curious, as Sue could make her way by herself from classroom to kitchen and back. It was not until we had been working for several months that she finally moved briefly across the open space, in a game of hide and seek.

It was increasingly evident that the actual movement experience was secondary to Sue's need for a relationship on her own terms—and her terms were primarily musical. She had nearly perfect tonal memory and regularly told me to sing specific words to specific tunes in specific rhythms. Sue made contact with the world, came "into the world," as it were, primarily through the medium of sound. Not such a strange position for a blind child. How, was the question, might Sue come "into the world" in her body, as well?

From that point movement was an accompaniment to singing, instead of the other way around. For example, with songs for support, Sue was able to explore and, perhaps, to define her body's size, comparing it to mine as we lay side-by-side on the couch to measure ourselves, accompanied by a song about "reaching our fingers and wiggling our toes." In addition, she began to test her strength by playing push and pull. We pushed sitting against each other, back-to back; we pushed and pulled, sitting at first, and later standing face-to-face. Eventually she began to experiment with stronger and more aggressive movements, such as stamping, kicking on the floor, and slapping the vinyl covers on the furniture. One day she told me she was "hiding." I found her and then she found me. This activity supported her understanding of object constancy much as "peek-a-boo" does for a sighted child. The game always produced some anxiety in Sue but it also brought about her first explorations of the unfamiliar space.

Sue called the kicking song "Bang Bang" and one day when she had asked for that tune and was lying on the floor, kicking and laughing, she suddenly asked for "Sue misses Mommy," the by now familiar song that usually went with holding hands and swaying or rocking. This time, however, she continued to kick, which prompted me to ask if she was "mad at Mommy for leaving?" She said nothing, but continued to kick and I changed the song to include the words "missing" and "mad." The new version stayed in our repertoire, along with the quieter rocking version.

After that day, Sue spent more session time with gross motor, percussive actions: stomping, punching and, at last with much persuasion, she ran albeit briefly, in the hall outside the therapy room. She was complimented for her bravery.

As long as she had singing for support, and was allowed to pick the song, Sue tried to do most of what was initiated. But she was rarely invested in any movement other than her flipping. It appeared that the flipping and the singing together formed Sue's defenses against much that was painful in her young life: the loss of her sister and grandmother to Texas and the suicide of her mother. Only once did she seem to be deeply involved in the movement, for its own sake. Toward the termination of our work, one day when we were rocking and singing "Sue misses Mommy," she seemed to "let go" and rock freely, lightly, and with her whole body. Perhaps, at last, a little of this child's grief had been released.

Sessions with Jon

From the outset, the sessions with Jon were very different from the sessions with Sue. He had worked with another dance/movement therapist and so did not have to ask, "What is movement?" In the classroom Jon had been reticent in the extreme. As soon as we came to the therapy room for the first session, it was clear that he remembered the room, furniture, and what to expect. To my surprise, in this special space he emerged, at least on the movement level, as an active and able child. He appeared "put together," where Sue seemed disconnected. All of his parts worked to form a whole. With the exception of his difficulty with direct, strong actions, Jon seemed to have what might be called a balance of movement qualities. His sense of himself in space was unusual for a blind child. He would do backward and forward somersaults in a continuous flowing sequence. His active joy in the movement experience was evident from the first moment.

But where was Jon's capacity for active joy when he was not in the movement room? The contrast between his manner in the classroom and the yard to his manner in our first session was so great that it required a reevaluation of this pliant, passive, nearly always obedient boy. Early on I had seen him as "happy in a secret world." In the movement session there was nothing secret about his pleasure. When other children, or his teacher, spoke to Jon, he smiled a vacant sort of smile. In our sessions he giggled and laughed aloud. But his difficulty with strong movements, coupled with his docility and his constant patting, seemed ample evidence that he had not found any productive outlet for his aggressive urges. All of this pointed to a direction for our work.

Another direction came from the fact that Jon's fluidity of movement was in sharp contrast to his attenuated language skills. Neither in class nor the movement room did he talk. Where language was a tool for Sue, for Jon language seemed, at best, a confused and private form of communication. Early in the morning on the day of our first session, I had come to the yard to tell Jon that later we were going to "do movement." He was by himself, patting on the fence, whispering, "flip, flip, flip." When I said, "Hi," he said, "Is gone." Trying to interpret his response, after a pause, I said, "If you want me to go away and you tell me to go, I will." He said, "I will go," and as I moved off, saying "Bye," he whispered "Bye," in return. This was typical of Jon's rare conversations.

There was, however, no difficulty when it came time for the session. He put his hand in mine and off we went. He took off his shoes without prompting and was ready for work. We explored the room together but I understood at once that he knew very well where he was. He did not initiate but willingly followed any movements I started. He responded verbally when directly asked to name his body and face parts, parroting the words I used but, interestingly, had trouble with "mouth."

Toward the end of the session, after we had gone through a wide range of movement actions, culminating with the backward somersaults, he sat on the floor and patted the carpet. As with Sue, I did the same, stopping and starting when he did. Unlike Sue, Jon made no comment and I began to think he would continue this "conversation" indefinitely. It was the teachers' practice to tell the children not to "flip," her word for all stereotyped behaviors. The teacher and I had talked about my intention to allow the behaviors during our session and she agreed that it might be meaningful in this special context. I stopped my patting part of the dialogue and told Jon that although he was not supposed to "flip" in the classroom, he could do so here in this room. Jon sat motionless for what seemed a long time. He then whispered, "Thank you," and, as if to test me, started to pat again. We patted until time for the session to close.

During the next few sessions, the focus was on Jon's impulse-driven patting motion. We patted body parts, knees, face, head, shoulders. We patted fast and slow, large and small, soft and loud. I accompanied with rhythmic chatter or little songs but, although he played all the patting games, Jon was silent except for giggles and an occasional repetition of a word. It was not surprising that he had difficulty with "loud." During our fourth session, Jon began to pat my face gently in an exploratory way, to find out who I was and, perhaps, to feel closer. After that he was more willing to follow noisy and aggressive movements such as slapping on the couch or pounding on the floor with our feet. In the pounding I discovered that he did not know how to make a fist. Making a fist and learning to punch occupied a good part of many subsequent sessions, and gradually, Jon was able to pound the carpet and punch the noisy couch.

The learning of these aggressive movements seemed to have an impact. On the day after our tenth session, Jon cried in anger for what was, according to his teacher, the first time. He had refused to eat his lunch and, in turn, his teacher refused to give him his favorite dessert. Jon began to cry and make growling noises. The teacher asked him to tell her he was "mad." He did repeat her words, obediently but without conviction. His tears were real, however, and so was the growl. Later that day the teacher said she viewed this "breakthrough" as a direct result of the dance/movement therapy. His anger, she said, was the most affect he had shown in the 5 years she had known him.

In a session the following day, Jon initiated a new activity: He climbed on my feet, holding on to my waist, and we rocked and turned, dancing while he hung on and giggled. The session continued to be especially playful until it was time to finish. He growled the same growl as the day before and volunteered, with little prompting, that he was "mad at Judith."

In all of the sessions to come, Jon utilized more strength and directness in his movements. He began to tease and use humor, as well. For example, when we sat on the floor, hands held, he would pull when I said push and push when I said pull, giggling while he did so. But he still would not talk to me, the teacher, or the other children except when under emotional stress, other than in the obedient echolalia observed earlier. At the end of each session, when told, "Well, Jon, it's time to go," he would echo, "Time to go." Then he would growl. One day I asked him, "Why are you mad?" not expecting an answer. He replied, "Because he goes 'grrr.'" This seemed to indicate confusion between the expression of the affect and the affect itself. He seemed to be telling me that he made the growl and was, therefore, angry, instead of the other way around. I told him I thought he made "grrr" because he was "mad at Judith for ending the session." I did not know what, if anything, he made of this exchange.

At the end of the following session, while we were putting on our shoes, I asked Jon if he remembered the previous session. "He said 'grrr!'" was his unexpected answer. At least he remembered and knew it was important.

In the weeks that remained before termination, Jon continued to expand his sense of himself, a sense that was nothing short of remarkable. He learned to jump over objects, to jump off the couch. He learned movement phrases: two hops, one jump, three slides, and the like. He made some progress in the expression of feelings, slapping the couch and growling at the end of sessions. He teased and giggled, joking through his movements.

When it came time to tell Jon that we were not going to be working together after the following week, I was aware of how attached to him I had become. After hearing that I would be going away, he patted a moment and then was absolutely still. I said it was hard, that I would miss him, too, but he would still be with his teacher at school and his family at home. Again he was still. Then he began to slap the couch as hard as he could with the full weight of his body. When I started to slap with him he took my hand at the wrist and slapped it on the couch as hard as he could, all the while making a crying noise, although no tears came. When I started to speak again, he patted my face and climbed into my lap and I sang a saying-good-bye song. After that we played some of our movement games: jumping, hopping, push and pulling, and he giggled as usual. At the end of the session, Jon crawled under the table and lay still; I did the same and for perhaps 5 minutes, the two of us were silent and motionless in the small, comforting shelter. The following week, after the final session with the two children, my notes read: Sue relates through sounds sent and received. Jon relates through his body and the modality of movement; it is his natural language.

Discussion and Conclusions

Of consequence for both children and, therefore, for the therapy, was the issue of their regression. Doctor M., an expert in the field, specifically stated in her notes that both Sue and Jon were "developing normally." But sometime around their second birthdays, both had lost considerable developmental ground. Why should this be so? An important clue lay in their bodies—specifically in their drive-discharge behaviors. Although Sue's flipping and Jon's patting were stylistically different, the purposes to which they were put can be considered the same. They were substitutes for more appropriate and useful outlets for aggression that become meaningfully socialized only through the medium of mobility. These two children gave first-hand evidence of Fraiberg's (1977) and Mittleman's (1954) theories. At an extraordinary developmental moment, they were denied a keystone to the future; they were denied mobility.

In any circumstance where movement or the inhibition of movement is so crucial, some form of therapeutic movement is indicated. But the techniques useful for these two were markedly different. Perhaps these differences should not have been surprising, given that Sue and Jon were in such different places with regard to the issues confronting the born blind: issues of self/nonself delineate, body image, language development, appropriate discharge of aggression, and the capacity to communicate accurately.

Sue seemed to delineate herself from others. She used pronouns correctly, knew everyone's name, had formed a relationship with her teacher and knew ways in which she could set about to meet some of her needs. She seemed to know what was real, even in the case of her mother's suicide, after the early denial was confronted. In the area of body image, she remained a puzzle: her movement was disjointed; there was no way to determine what her shoes represented to her. At the outset of therapy, Sue seemed to use words as her chief form of communication. But when looking at her body and its movement, would one have judged her communications to be accurately representing her?

If one considers the integration of an individual's body and its general movement, together with the person's language and general mode of behavior—in other words, a "sense" of the integration of the individual's parts as a measure of the accuracy of their communications—then Sue did not accurately represent herself in her verbal dialogue. Her body, with its intense, impulse-driven behaviors and stiff, disjointed look, did not express the same message as her far superior language ability. It was not by words that the signal was given that she was in mourning. And it was only when her words were joined with movement expression, mediated by song, that she was able to work through her sorrow.

With Jon, the distinction between self and other and the relationship to external reality were less clear. He did not have a strong relationship with his teacher; he did not usually use correct pronouns, referring to himself as "he," and he seldom used proper names. It was not clear if he perceived himself as a whole separate individual, as evidenced further by his possible confusion over cause and effect. Yet his movements indicated another aspect of him, just as Sue's had, that might otherwise have been missed.

It was clear from the outset that Jon's communications were body oriented and his dialogue a movement dialogue. Nothing in Jon's history provided an explanation for this; he seemed in his body and its movement, a sort of natural phenomenon. Unfortunately, the language of the body and movement are a foreign language in most of the places Jon had found himself. If Jon's "native language," as it were, could be understood, then one could see the potential for him to become a more integrated human being. Despite his massive handicap, Jon's movement picture was not one in which any major ingredients were missing. In our short time together, he had come a distance in expressing aggression, in expressing himself in a fuller way. But if Jon was to function and mature in the world at large, he certainly needed to learn the words—the language of his fellows, those able in sight, perhaps less so in movement.

Because both children used stereotyped movements, it was not difficult to begin to form a relationship by mirroring or reflecting back their particular ideosyncratic patterns. With Sue it was equally, if not more important, to meet her where she was in the world of music. After the initial relationship, the therapeutic task with both children was to add or create the missing ingredient. In the most immediate terms, Sue needed to find a way to mourn and Jon needed to get mad and to assert himself. Our movement work seemed to help in both these areas.

In terms of long-range prospects, the situation was more troubling. Jon's obvious communication problems would be hard to overcome. As for Sue, although she may have been more advanced in certain ways, her inability to integrate her words with her real feelings presaged, at best, a fragmented dialogue.

When I came to work with Sue and Jon, they were 7 years old. Intervention on the movement level would have been more meaningful if it had begun much earlier. Barraga (1976) writes:

The extent to which vision is actually a stimulating and facilitating factor in affective, psychomotor, perceptual and cognitive development is not known....If there is a strong interrelationship between movement and learning, then for the children who are blind, movement may be the most accurate replacement for vision for clarifying information about the world. Perhaps physical movement alone, if carefully designed, could facilitate the same quality of psychomotor development as that achieved by children who have both vision and movement. (pp. 25–26)

Sue and Jon did not have an early enough intervention to provide a remedy for the many difficulties caused by their blindness. They were fortunate to be in a fine facility and were responsive to the movement experience.

Regarding children born blind, Fraiberg (1976) writes:

Everything we do to create a pleasurable sensation in the body ego itself, which must precede the sense of self, is going to enhance the body image on a primitive level and will perhaps begin the progress toward "I"...There is enough evidence to show that this is one place where we can effectively intervene, that the building of self-image begins with the building of body image, and therefore all that we can do in early intervention...to enhance the body self will presumably show up in the enhancement of self. (p. 158)

Certainly, an earlier opportunity might have made a significant difference for these two children.

For the therapist there are certain frustrations with this population when intervention on the movement level is as delayed as it was with Sue and Jon. The satisfactions from the work need to be in the small, subtle evidence of possible growth, and in the insights that arise from close, ongoing contact with so unique a population.

12

Sandra: The Case of an Adopted Sexually Abused Child

Steve Harvey

When a child is adopted at an age beyond infancy, the child's ability to develop a trusting parent–child relationship is particularly difficult. McNamara and McNamara (1990) point out that by the time older children reach an adoptive home, they have often experienced many foster care placements and repeated separations from caregivers. In addition, these children may have suffered abuse or neglect in their earlier families. Despite adoptive parents' best efforts, such children may perceive all adults as threatening and unprotective. And because of the lack of any trusting relationship, such children are often unable to resolve earlier traumatic experiences and, thus, are at high risk of developing major difficulties as they mature. Clearly, an important goal of any intervention is to help such children learn to trust.

This chapter presents the case study of a girl who was sexually assaulted by her birth parents. It recounts the therapeutic work done with her and her family over a period of 2 1/2 years.

Controversies Involving Sexual Abuse of Young Children

McNamara (1989) estimates that by the time foster care children reach school age, approximately three out of four have experienced some form of sexual abuse. As most children keep the abuse secret, a child's social history may be misleading.

Certain past adoption practices encouraged both adoptive parents and adoptive children not to deal with the children's histories. Johnson (1988), McNamara (1989), and Ryan (1989), point out that the practice of avoiding past issues can have significant negative consequences in the adoptive family. Young children who have been sexually abused prior to their adoptive placement experience ongoing feelings of betrayal and mistrust. Such feelings can be awakened in children even as they experience close physical contact with their adoptive parents. Further, discomforting emotional closeness and intimacy may easily lead to acting-out behaviors, such as aggression and even sexual perpetration on younger children.

Given these potential difficulties, clearly it is important for families adopting young, sexually abused children to deal with the victimization. Ryan (1989, 1990) suggests that family-oriented therapy is imperative. However, such family therapy is not without its difficulties. Although many children may have been sexually assaulted, others have not. Therapists working with young children need to be particularly aware that their clients are extremely vulnerable to influence from adults (parents as well as therapists) and may produce statements in order to meet adult expectations.

Therapists then, need to address issues of sexual abuse carefully so as not to generate false information. At the same time, without addressing past abuse in a complete way, the development of trust is unlikely.

The creative-arts therapies offer a valuable modality in which these concerns can be addressed. Although the words of child and parent do need to be considered, the expressive-arts therapies can engage both in joint activities that facilitate their emotional expressiveness and interaction without reliance on language. The power of the arts is such that the child can be helped without a detailed discussion of the child's history.

As young children begin to trust their new parents, they may also begin to identify past episodes of abuse. These disclosures are a by-product, rather than a direct goal of the therapy process. The creative-arts therapist can leave the direct investigations of sexual abuse to other professionals. This strategy was followed in the following case study, in which a 3 $^1/_2$-year-old girl presented symptoms suggestive of sexual abuse. Such issues were not addressed by direct questioning but after approximately a year of intervention spent improving mother–child and family–child interactions, the child made unprompted statements to a social service evaluator who later confirmed sexual assault. In this way, the process of therapy and evaluation were able to be kept separate.

A number of authors report on activities that are meaningful for the creative-arts therapist working with family interventions. A summary of some of the work relevant to this discussion follows.

Molding and Interactive Synchrony

Meekums (1991), describing movement games used to improve mother–child interactions in families at risk for child abuse, specifically looks at interactions called "molding" and "interactive synchrony." Molding refers to the way parents' and childrens' body shapes fit into and around each other. Interactive synchrony refers to their movements that involve changes in gestures or postures that begin and end at the same time. An increase in both molding and interactive synchrony is associated with improved parent–child relationships. Meekums' interventions include interactive dances and movement developed for children and their mothers. These structured activities are used as a way to observe problems and at the same time create change.

Attachment and Attunement

The development of positive attachment and emotional communication between adoptive parents and children is particularly challenging in the event of sexual abuse prior to adoption. Attachment refers to the emotional tie between parent and child that makes them important to each other. The tie grows out of a pattern of adult–child interactions and rests on the development of expectations as to how the adult provides comfort and protection when the child feels distressed, overwhelmed, or frightened. Such parent behaviors include (a) sensitivity to nonverbal communication; (b) physical availability; and (c) attunement, that is, nonverbal matching of emotional communication. Nonverbal communication patterns between parent and child are especially important. Ainsworth, Blehar, Waters, and Hall (1978) and Romer and Sossin (1990) stress that the parents' abilities to touch and hold their child, especially when the child is distressed during the early months of life, contribute to later patterns of intimate relationships.

In preschool years, children enter into what Bowlby (1980) calls a "goal-correcting relationship" with their caretakers. In this phase, children are able to cooperate and negotiate even when they are distressed. Interaction is characterized by an ability to engage in mutual problem-solving, some role reversal (i.e., the ability to identify with the significant other's role), and development of empathy. In movement activities, such as follow-the-leader, or in dramatic storytelling, children at this stage are able to exchange roles and pay attention to their parents' actions as well as their own. Children with insecure attachments have great difficulty with such cooperative interaction at this stage and are avoidant, resistant, or disorganized in their behavior.

Stern (1977, 1985, 1990) introduces a concept closely related to attachment, called "affective attunement." Based on observations of interactive communication and narrative storytelling, Stern discusses the importance of the development of empathy and emotional understanding between parent and child. Such understanding initially develops out of nonverbal communication in which parents and infants match both body and vocal rhythms when communicating strong feelings. Such matching can occur simultaneously or develop in a turn-taking fashion. One member of the parent–child dyad expresses a strong feeling through body or vocal rhythms, which in turn triggers the other to match or "attune to" the same feeling. This shared rhythmic emotional expression later influences narrative play. Thus, how a parent attunes to a child's early expressions has a strong impact on the child's later experience of emotion. Without the development of rhythmic matching, a child's capacity for empathy and ability to share feelings is compromised at the body level. Taken together, this research suggests that a child's early interactive experience with caretakers has a strong impact on all of the child's later interactions.

Case Study

Mr. and Mrs. Robinson were referred for expressive therapy with Sandra, their 3 ½-year-old foster-adoptive daughter, shortly after Sandra was placed with them. Sandra came to her new parents from a program for children who had been removed from their birth parents due to abuse and neglect and were to be permanently placed in new homes. Two months after Sandra was placed with the Robinsons, she was referred for therapy by a social worker.

In the initial interview, Mrs. Robinson described a number of difficulties. Sandra constantly moved and talked and ignored almost all verbal direction. She woke up two or three times a night and was unable to go back to sleep for several hours. She masturbated in front of her parents and other children and stopped only when Mrs. Robinson picked her up, held her, and removed her from the room. Sandra had confided in Mrs. Robinson that other unnamed adults had touched her "pee-pee." When Sandra did play, however, she could entertain herself for hours without seeming to need adult attention or socialization with other children. Sandra was described as talking nonstop and had several imaginary friends.

Sandra was a blond-haired, brown-eyed girl of average height with a slight build. During our first conversation, she changed the subject so often it was hard to follow her. When she began to play with the toys, she shifted rapidly from one to another without completing any play ideas. As she played, her body movements quickened and she did not recuperate with physical stops or rest points. When Mrs. Robinson tried to play with Sandra, the child ignored her, shifting her focus to another activity. Little eye contact was observed between the two, and Sandra kept turning her body away from Mrs. Robinson.

I told Mrs. Robinson that I would like to watch the two of them at play. My intention was to outline repetitive interactive patterns between Sandra and her mother and to identify areas for change, the change to be accomplished by developing new games to focus on the interactive difficulties that Mrs. Robinson and I agreed were present.

Initial Observations: "The Chase"

In the following three sessions, Sandra and her adoptive mother were asked to complete movement games, dramatic play, and a series of drawing activities. The games included follow-the-leader and a mirroring activity, and both Sandra and her mother were to take turns leading. In dramatic play and art activities, Sandra and Mrs. Robinson first drew or played together. Mrs. Robinson was asked to leave for approximately 5 minutes and was then reintroduced into the activity. Comparisons of their initial interaction, the individual and the reunion play were useful in determining the influence the adoptive mother had on Sandra.

During both mirroring and follow-the-leader, Sandra became very distracted, darting quickly from one part of the room to another. She was unable to take turns and did not allow Mrs. Robinson to lead. Mrs. Robinson was able to engage her daughter fleetingly only by following Sandra's movements. Sandra made very little eye contact and did not adjust either the shape of her body or rhythm of her movements to allow for mutual activity. After several darting movements around the room, Sandra became more and more excited about leaving Mrs. Robinson behind. This resembled a game of "chase," rather than follow-the-leader and Mrs. Robinson was frustrated after a few minutes of trying to redirect Sandra verbally. No positive feelings showed from either mother or daughter and the only result was that Sandra gained physical distance from Mrs. Robinson.

Sandra's behavior was similar when she and her mother were provided with props (several large stuffed animals, stretch ropes, parachutes, dolls, and pillows). Sandra did not develop any dramatic play, but moved through the room from object to object in the same way as before. When her mother left the room briefly and when she returned, Sandra's behavior was unaffected. She continued to use the props to escalate her physical activity in an excitable, non-stop fashion. This behavior underlined Sandra's inability to sustain any mutual give-and-take relationship and seemed to indicate a marked lack of healthy attachment.

During the second session, Sandra was asked to draw, while her mother sat next to her. She drew two geometric shapes, which she identified as a man and a little girl. Both drawings, within the developmental range of a 3 1/2 year old, suggested that Sandra had the ability to represent herself with another, signifying some relatedness. Sandra did not represent herself with a female figure, however, which may have reflected her difficulty in attaching to her adoptive mother. Sandra was asked to draw again when her mother moved to the other side of the room. The second drawing was significantly different. Sandra was unable to complete any figures and began scribbling in a disorganized way. This difference suggested that Sandra may have been able to use her 6 months of placement to organize a rudimentary concept of relationship, but only when her mother was nearby.

In the next session, given the choice of drawing or physical play with her mother, Sandra chose drawing. They were asked to draw a family. After a brief time, Sandra made high-pitched noises that turned to screams. She scribbled over the picture she and her mother had made together and then tore it up. Despite many suggestions from her mother and myself, Sandra was unable to return to this activity in any constructive way and needed to be calmed down.

In the following session, I met with Mrs. Robinson to outline the problems that seemed to stand in the way of Sandra's development of a more trusting relationship. The difficulties included: (a) Sandra's inability to stay focused on her adoptive mother; (b) her difficulty with taking turns; (c) her tendency to develop physical activity that was more intense than the activities with her mother; (d) her inability to approach her adoptive mother; and (e) their mutual inability to use shaping or matching of bodies while in interaction. The result was a pattern of nonverbal communication that made the sharing of emotional caring, protection, or safety unlikely.

These observations helped to establish initial treatment goals: (a) to assist Sandra in learning to take turns in both movement and drawing activities; (b) to enable Sandra to generate her own expressive movement and graphic ideas, while in contact with her mother; (c) to help Sandra spontaneously approach Mrs. Robinson; and (d) to help Mrs. Robinson recognize Sandra's nonverbal expressions as they occurred and to respond to them so as to build mutual activity of longer duration. The central idea was to help the adoptive mother and her child develop play that enabled an exchange of genuine feelings. Once interaction could be established through games, the goal would be to help Sandra and her adoptive parents express deeper feelings. For Sandra, these feelings involved both adoption and abuse; for her parents, emotional support and protection. Without first achieving some change in interaction, there was little likelihood that emotional sharing, necessary for the development of trust, would occur. After changes were achieved in therapy sessions, goals would then be to assist Sandra and her adoptive parents in making such changes at home.

Sandraland and Momland

In the first series of play activities, Sandra and her mother created a "Sandraland" and a "Momland" on which either could sit, stand, or move. The lands were made of two 5-by-2 pillows, about 10 feet apart. This separation seemed to enable Sandra to respond to her mother. Although both mother and child were on their respective lands, they followed each other's movements, gestures, and body postures. The mirroring activities were broadened; Sandra or Mrs. Robinson made a face, then a gesture, then a body shape to show feelings such as anger, happiness, fear, or sadness—while the other followed in a playful manner. When Mrs. Robinson and Sandra were in these defined spaces, activities were far more successful and lasted up to several minutes without verbal direction from an adult. While at some distance from her mother, Sandra was more able to create movement ideas for her mother to follow, and she was more ready to respond to her mother's ideas, as well.

Over several weeks of this game, Sandra and Mrs. Robinson appeared able, for brief periods, to share a feeling of genuine caring for each other in a playful way. Occasionally, Sandra became so engaged in her mother's movements that she ran to "Momland" where Mrs. Robinson greeted her with a hug. Sandra's mother reported that this was the first time they had been able to play together and "have fun." Thus, a starting place was provided for Sandra to experience an adult in a positive way. She did not always have to run away in order to control her feelings.

As Sandra continued to share positive feelings with her mother, she added more choices: going to "Momland," going back to her own "land," and selecting props that showed a variety of feelings. Sandra's movement back and forth became more elaborate as she developed styles of running, skipping, and crawling. After several weeks, Sandra climbed into her mother's lap for short periods of time. When this happened, both the mother's and child's bodies began to adapt to the shape of each other more easily, which in turn produced a more positive holding behavior. Sandra appeared to enjoy these brief moments before she would once again run quickly back to her own "land."

Holding Homework

At this point, holding and rocking activities were suggested as homework. The goal was to help Sandra and her mother generalize the gains made in the sessions. Sandra's mother was asked to hold Sandra in her lap and rock her but Sandra was resistant and began to complain and struggle.

When she reported this, I told Mrs. Robinson to continue holding Sandra lightly, in a soothing manner, to increase her hold when Sandra's physical resistance increased and to relax her hold when Sandra relaxed. Sandra was encouraged to breathe deeply during the holding activities in order to decrease her muscular tension. One of the goals was to help Sandra and her mother become aware of kinesthetic and touch cues, to adjust their movement patterns to each other in mutually responsive ways. After some practice, Sandra was able to use her mother's light touches to help her relax. After several weeks of practice, Sandra and Mrs. Robinson exhibited the kind of holding commonly seen in securely attached infants during their first year. Both mother and child enjoyed these shared moments and their mutual sensitivity to changes in one another's tension flow while in close physical contact enabled Mrs. Robinson and Sandra to experience attunement.

Tug-of-War

Soon after the touch and holding activity became enjoyable, Sandra introduced a new idea. She suggested that when she was on her own island and her mother on "Mom Island," the two of them would use the parachute or bungee cord to have a tug-of-war. Sandra was able to sustain long periods of eye contact and high intensity pulling while also having fun with her mother. After some weeks, Sandra introduced a frightening ghost/monster into the game. When Sandra played with this image, she showed genuine fear. After the introduction of this imaginary character, the first of many games were developed that included the theme of "being safe."

Chasing Away the Ghost

With the help of scarves and pieces of cloth, I physicalized the ghost/monster. Sandra and her mother developed dances that included stomping, clapping, singing, and blowing motions to chase the ghost away. The game was elaborated as Sandra and Mrs. Robinson rehearsed. After some practice, I approached the mother and daughter with a "ghost scarf" while the pair performed dances to chase the ghost away. At one point, Sandra excitedly wanted the ghost to fly out of the room. Through the repetition of the game, Mrs. Robinson and Sandra began to use similar gestures and postures to accomplish their task. Their movements were matched with songs about the ghost's departing. In this game, Sandra and her mother developed a metaphor with which to address Sandra's underlying fears and her need for protection. Clearly, the sharing of movement patterns in the holding, rocking, and tug-of-war activities were now being extended into more elaborate dances. Sandra and her mother were increasing their connection to each other.

Adoption Island

After 2 months of treatment, Sandra's adoptive father was invited to join the therapy. In the next three sessions, the island game was expanded to include "New Family Island" and "Old Family Island." Stuffed animals were put on the Old Family Island to represent Sandra's birth family. Sandra and her adoptive parents were encouraged to introduce dance variations in which they moved back and forth between these two family locations. At times, the parents would swing or carry Sandra from one family island to the other. On other occasions, Sandra and the Robinsons had "races" from one place to the other. These races were elaborated using slow motion or backward racing with each family member contributing. During the races, Sandra and her parents began to enjoy each other and suggested new movement ideas to keep the game going. Feelings about leaving the old family and being in a new family were discussed during this activity.

These games provided another metaphor by which the family began to develop a more trusting relationship. As each person contributed to the movement and the drama, they expressed, identified, and resolved many relationship issues in a playful manner. This method of expressing an emotional issue was particularly useful for Sandra. She was deeply involved in the drama of leaving her old family and joining her new family. After a period of these activities, Sandra demonstrated a visible shift from the more fearful defensive feelings she initially presented to more active engagement and security. Although she did not discuss the complex issues centered on separation, termination of parental rights, and the new attachments of adoption, Sandra's body movement and play seemed to help her approach these issues in a real and meaningful way.

Initial Disclosures

Following the series of sessions in which Sandra showed more positive feelings toward both her adoptive parents, she told her mother that she had been sexually assaulted by her biological parents. In the following session, without prompting, Sandra drew a figure she identified as her birth father touching her "pee-pee." She drew a penis in the genital area of the birth father, birth mother, and a little girl figure. As she drew, Sandra became extremely agitated. She hit the figures, scribbled over them, and eventually tore up the drawings.

Sandra's disclosures were duly reported but during the ensuing interview with the authorities, she denied any sexual abuse. Directly after the interview, however, Sandra told her adoptive mother that she had lied to the interviewers. It is important to note that Sandra, her adoptive mother and father, and I had not talked about issues of sexual abuse through the previous 9 months of treatment. The interventions had been directed, as stated above, toward increasing interaction and playfulness. All activities had been developed using Sandra's cues. In this way, the treatment issues were kept separate from evaluation issues.

It is important to remember that young children often initiate disclosures about their pasts only to retract them before finally make more complete, spontaneous statements (Summit, 1983; Waterman, Kelly, McCord,& Olivieri, 1990). Although the therapeutic strategy had been to improve play interaction, enhance sharing of emotional content, and increase the development of affective attunement, the assumption had been that disclosures would proceed at Sandra's own pace.

Return of "The Chase"

In the two sessions following Sandra's interview with the authorities, she wanted to play a "chasing the monster—go away game" with her mother helping her. The game was finally finished when Sandra buried the monster in pillows and she and her mother held hands and jumped on the spot. Sandra was less playful during this game and showed more focused concern. Some fearfulness returned. This repetitive play suggested that Sandra had found a symbolic expression of her fear, but was not yet able to find a positive resolution.

During the next several sessions, Sandra reverted to the interactions she had shown in her initial visits. When mother or father suggested ideas or got physically close to her, she darted off, playing "chase" again. Sandra stopped contributing her own ideas to their activities. The adoptive parents became frustrated, and gave Sandra commands such as, "Stop! Come back! Complete this!" But their orders only added to Sandra's distancing activities. No empathy, emotional understanding, or compassion seemed available between the parents and their child during this time.

In order to help the family focus, I asked Sandra and her parents to draw together. The activity was videotaped. As Sandra drew, her parents tried to guide her drawings with suggestions, but their comments agitated and distracted Sandra. Despite their best intentions, The Robinsons' interaction with Sandra only had negative results.

During the next session, the parents were shown the video. As their comments were discussed with them, the Robinsons were able to observe how their controlling interactions inhibited their daughter's expression of feelings. After this time, both mother and father became more supportive and their relationship with Sandra improved.

Mother's Touch: A Safehouse

Following the disclosures of abuse, Sandra's nightmares and agitated behavior returned for several months. At this point, the father was no longer in the sessions. The primary focus now was to help Sandra see Mrs. Robinson as a protective figure. A secondary goal was to encourage the development of greater intimacy. Activities included having Sandra and her mother use the pillows to make a "safehouse" into which no monster or ghost could enter. More holding was also included in sessions and the holding was elaborated with games in which Mrs. Robinson rolled Sandra in the pillows, or Sandra rolled and turned on large pillows called "Mom's lap."

During holding times, Sandra's mother was again encouraged to touch Sandra in order to recognize her tension flow patterns. She was asked to verbalize the feelings Sandra seemed to be expressing and to reassure Sandra that she was safe. Throughout these holds, Sandra yelled that she was being hurt or tortured despite the relatively light touch used by her mother. Sandra also made these comments while rolling on the "lap" pillows. Intimacy with her adoptive mother appeared to stimulate flashbacks or a physical reliving of the trauma associated with the sexual abuse of her earlier life. The holding continued for approximately 2 months with less and less time needed before Sandra calmed down and relaxed in her mother's lap or on the pillows.

Sandra and her mother also developed closeness while moving through space using a stretch rope to physically connect them. There was also a stretch blanket that covered Sandra and her mother's entire bodies. Inside this blanket, when one person moved, the blanket naturally helped the other move, as well. Both Mrs. Robinson and Sandra became interested in making shapes with their bodies while using both these props. For the first time, Sandra and her mother spontaneously showed true shaping over extended periods of time.

Sandra and Mrs. Robinson then extended the theme of a safehouse. They made drawings of monsters behind protective walls or in jail and developed stories involving monsters who could not hurt younger, more vulnerable children. Mother figures were included in protective ways. Sandra and her mother made tape recordings of these stories and Sandra listened to the stories at night as she was falling asleep. As Sandra and her mother became more invested and engaged in all of the metaphors involving safety and protection, Sandra began to spend more time close to Mrs. Robinson's body.

Verbal Disclosure: The More Complete Story

During this phase of treatment, which lasted four to 4–5 months, Sandra described past abuse and then chose a safe game to play with her mother. Often

Sandra became afraid after talking about the abuse and asked Mrs. Robinson to hold her.

All the sexual assaults by both her birth mother and father described by Sandra occurred in the bathtub. Sandra reported that other adults were also involved. She spoke of threats, including kidnap and murder, to keep her from revealing these secrets. Sandra also reported being left alone in a room and given only dog or cat food to eat. During this period of disclosures, Sandra compulsively masturbated at school and at home; in front of her peers or family. She also began to ask other children at her day-care center to touch her sexually. Nightmares returned. Finally, just before her fifth birthday, Sandra reported her abuse fully to a Department of Social Services worker. After the interview, Sandra used the "Chase Away the Monster" game to help reduce her anxiety. She completed this game, adding several new versions in a dance with her mother to chase the monster/ghost away. Sandra and Mrs. Robinson both experienced intense feelings during this enactment. Sandra again was fearful, and Mrs. Robinson was focused, intent, and serious when dancing away the monsters.

Getting the "Bugs" Out

Following the disclosures and ensuing development of compulsive masturbation, nightmares, and sleeping difficulties, Sandra was asked if she could describe her feelings. She said it felt like "bugs inside." From this, she and her mother together developed the idea of making dances to "get the bugs out." After creating a dance in a therapy session, Sandra and her mother were given a homework assignment: to spend approximately 20 minutes every day on their dance. The therapy sessions that followed were videotaped and Sandra and her mother were then told to watch the dances at home and come up with movement elaborations.

Both Mrs. Robinson and Sandra contributed ideas for their dance, small movements of fingers or facial expressions, as well as larger arm and whole-body gestures. It was significant that during this dance development, Sandra was highly cooperative with Mrs. Robinson. Also, she spontaneously wanted to match her mother's rhythm for longer periods of time. This marked the first time in treatment that Sandra seemed to generate a secure attachment style for extended periods of time without an adult's direction.

During a later attempt at an in-session "bug dance," while Sandra was being the leader, she bounced her buttocks on the floor, saying that the bugs were in her vagina. At this point, the dance was stopped and I suggested that we needed a "bug trap" and directed Sandra to sit on her mother's lap and kick a pillow (to engage her lower body). Kicking the pillow was called "Putting the bugs in the trap." After a few kicks, Sandra's kicking and yelling became rageful. She continued to kick and make loud noises. She then added pushing and hitting, as well as kicking to her effort.

In the next session, I introduced fast and slow music so that Sandra could become even more involved in elaborating her bug dance. Through several weeks, Sandra changed her bug dancing to match changes in the music, sometimes slow music from the classical repertoire, and sometimes jazz. During the homework assignment, Sandra was asked to observe when her movement was following the music and when it was not. It took several video observation sessions for Sandra to identify with her own movement. Once she was able to observe her own movements, she actively made choices in how to move, developing control over her body.

After approximately 3 months of various versions of "bug dancing," Sandra introduced further elaborations, such as choosing different pillows to dance on or around, different spatial arrangements, different pieces of music using different rhythms, and the like. Sandra also elaborated on her dramatic imagery and used the new imagery in her dances. With this development, her mother was able to sit and watch while Sandra danced her "bugs" out for longer periods. This phase of therapy ended when Sandra identified herself as a cocoon, and changed into a butterfly as she emerged from under buried pillows and slowly extended her arms to her full kinesphere, saying she could now fly to her mother. These expressions were deeply moving for Mrs. Robinson. For the first time, the adoptive mother could witness her daughter approach her completely. As with the other dances, this piece was videotaped and Sandra and her mother were eager to show the tape to her father and describe the related steps.

Learning How to Dance Good-bye

During this part of the therapy, Sandra's father again joined sessions so that Sandra could show him her bug dances. He appreciated and more deeply understood his daughter's feelings about her past victimization. These final visits stretched over approximately another 6 months, with Sandra being seen every other week. During sessions, Sandra and her mother chose which games they wanted to play. Their new enactments were compared with the videos of previous games from almost 2 $\frac{1}{2}$ years of treatment. Sandra was able to talk about how the dances and games had changed.

Sandra continued to have occasional difficulties in her chosen activities, such as Monster/Ghost, Safehouse, or mutual drawings. Both she and her mother were able to identify these times and take corrective action. For example, they were able to change the content of the games so that Sandra could plan how she, or a representation of herself, could be safe. Once, when she acted out a story of a little girl who was lost and could not find her way home, she was able to draw a map. On another occasion, she drew a house where she wasn't lonely and a map of how to get there as well. Using this map drawing, Sandra created a dance about how to find her new mother.

To end therapy, Sandra was asked to choose her favorite activity and develop a goodbye ritual. Sandra chose making a "safehouse." We spent several sessions in preparing. Sandra and Mrs. Robinson made a house out of pillows together and spent time inside retelling stories of their therapy activities: chasing away the ghost, making bug dances. Finally, in the last session, Sandra invited me into the house to say goodbye. At this time, I told Sandra how much I would miss her. Then we all agreed that she and her mother had learned many dances and games to play by themselves. Though we might be sad, we could remember each other by playing the games we had developed together.

Summary

Therapy was terminated approximately 2 $\frac{1}{2}$ years after it had begun. The relationship between adoptive parents and child had clearly changed. Both parents, especially Sandra's mother, could truly assume more protective and nurturant roles. In turn, Sandra was able to feel close to Mr. and Mrs. Robinson. She was also able to disclose episodes of previous abuse and experience posttraumatic flashbacks. Her adoptive parents were able to participate protectively in dramatic metaphors of this trauma through the various games we had developed. Finally, on a movement level, Sandra and her adoptive parents were able to develop a matching in their interactions, and some sense of calmness and relaxation with physical closeness.

This case study illustrates how expressive-arts therapy can help children and their parenting figures develop organized expression and use that expression to share the deep emotions necessary for the development of trust and attachment.

13

Early Intervention with Children at Risk for Attachment Disorders

Bette Blau and Debra Reicher

"Attachment" is a term that received increasing attention following John Bowlby's systematic inquiry into the effects of early separation of mother and child and the ensuing effects on the child's personality (Mahler, 1970; Stern, 1985).[1] The term attachment captures the central importance of a parent–child relationship and its impact on the child's subsequent development. Attachment has become generalized to numerous theoretical perspectives, all of which share a common focus on the bonding process between caregiver and child (Mahler, 1970; Stern, 1985; Winnicott, 1965).

Bowlby (1980) writes that the infant exhibits three different responses to separation from the primary caregiver—protest, despair, and detachment. He also points out that the loss of and/or separation from a mother figure has a far greater impact on a young child than had been earlier presumed. He adds that "the young child's hunger for his mother's love and presence is as great as his hunger for food" (Bowlby, 1980, p. xiii).

The basic premise of this chapter is twofold: that infancy is a highly significant developmental period and that the patterns of child behavior and caregiving established during infancy provide a foundation for the child's future relationships and self-concept.

The most important factor in the formation of healthy attachment and subsequent separation are the multisensory, affective, and motor interactions that occur between parent and infant. Individuals respond to a wide range of nonverbal signals. Facial expressions, voice qualities, movements, and touch— all can convey feelings of anger, impatience, pleasure, or ambivalence. These signals are used consciously and unconsciously by parents when communicating with their infants and the infants are active participants in the interaction. For example, mothers instinctively raise the pitch of their voices, open their eyes wide and bob their heads when speaking to an infant. In turn, infants respond with a wide range of body movements, smiles and gurgles that encourage the mother to continue. A baby may try to elicit a response from a withdrawn, stone-faced mother by engaging in a series of body movements, facial expressions, and sounds. If the mother remains emotionally unavailable, the infant may withdraw all efforts to stimulate a response (Toda & Fogel, 1993). If parents are continually tense, the baby will feel the tension.

Infants experience the environment through channels that are often out of the adult's conscious awareness. Signs and signals that are received by infants include changes in body movements such as touch, equilibrium, posture, tension, and rhythm; and changes in voice quality such as tempo, pitch, vibration, and tone (Spitz, 1965). Because emotions affect both body movements and voice quality, caregivers need to be aware of their own feelings, the feelings their babies engender in them, and the degree of impact that movements and voice quality have on their children.

Infants do not possess sophisticated methods for dealing with environmental demands. Their bodies are the vehicles through which they cope and adapt to both internal and external stimuli. For example, an infant sucks his thumb in a self-soothing effort to relieve tension; he turns his head away when no longer hungry; and averts his gaze in order to avoid overstimulation. Caregivers need to be able to respond empathetically to such nonverbal communications. Some parents benefit from special training that focuses on sensitizing them to their children's needs. The parent's success in picking up and sensitively responding to the child's cues is important if the child is to move successfully from one stage of development to the next.

Cycles of infant/caregiver interactions that are repetitive and consistent create an emotional climate within which the baby gradually transforms meaningless stimuli into meaningful signals. It is not any particular interaction but the pattern of all of the moments together that helps to determine how the child will develop. If the infant/caregiver interaction is repeatedly ineffective, it is difficult for the child to develop a coherent, organized view of the world or a sense of emotional well-being.

The following are three examples of risks for impaired mother/infant communication that often provoke subsequent problems: (1) children who are predisposed to developmental difficulties; (2) caregivers who have significant levels of psychopathology; and (3) parent/child dyads that are temperamentally mismatched.

Children born with a wide range of developmental problems may not have the "sending power" needed to make their signs and signals easily understood. For example, a premature infant with an underdeveloped nervous system may not be able to regulate stimuli, and may, as a result, be hyperexcitable. Babies born with cerebral palsy may exhibit behaviors and affects that appear chaotic or rigid. Infants with low muscle tone can appear apathetic and withdrawn. In addition, there are babies born with unusual sensitivities (Bergman & Escalona, 1949) and/or unusual drive endowments (Alpert & Neubauer, 1956) due to constitutional or hereditary factors. Such infants may withdraw from touch, exhibit exaggerated startle responses or appear as hypo- or hyperaggressive. Parents' feelings of inadequacy associated with having a "less than perfect child" often interfere with their abilities to read and sensitively respond to their infant's cues. Such parents are particularly in need of appropriate help.

The following vignettes offer examples of the problems in the three categories of risk cited previously. First, an infant who is born blind poses significant challenges to the caregiver.

> A blind 4 month old ceases all activity, becoming very still when his mother approaches. He does not vocalize, reach for, or turn toward her. He invests all of his anticipatory excitement and energy in attending to the sounds and odors associated with his mother's approach. Mother mistakes his quiet intensity for apathy and emotional distance. She feels rejected, believing that her baby doesn't love her. She, in turn, withdraws from the very contact so desperately needed—the tactile, kinesthetic and vocal stimulation which can help her blind child feel loved and foster his ability to organize his world. The reciprocal mother-child interaction has been short-circuited as a result of the misreading of a baby's cues. (Blau, 1989, p. 2)

Second, a caregiver with significant pathology and/or unresolved issues in his/her family of origin is at risk for having an impaired ability to respond appropriately and sensitively to an infant. Such parents often respond out of their own needs as opposed to the needs of the infant.

The following briefly describes the behavior of Sally, a mother of a 10-month-old boy. Sally's own mother had not encouraged her to be autonomous;

as a child, she had not been allowed to play outdoors or "get dirty." She had been "forced" to take dance lessons and was viewed by her mother as the "pretty little girl." Sally grew up believing she existed to meet her mother's needs.

> When interacting with her 10-month-old boy, Sally is alternately rejecting and overstimulating, depending upon her own mood. She finds it difficult to allow her child the autonomy to engage in spontaneous, exploratory behavior. She insists on his playing with objects "the right way"—her way, or not at all. She is often stifling and intrusive. Her controlling behavior blocks the initiative and spontaneity of her child's "true self." The development of autonomy and self-esteem is thwarted as a result of the parent responding to her own needs rather than to those of her child. (Blau, 1989, p. 2)

Finally, a parent and infant may be temperamentally "mismatched."

> Twelve month old Molly is a quiet subdued, passive child. Her mother is an energetic, active woman who continually stimulates Molly by placing toys in front of her, tickling her and maintaining a constant stream of quick, staccato-like chatter. Molly, overwhelmed by her mother's "typical" behavior, initially averts eye gaze and finally moves to a corner with her back facing her mother. (Reicher, 1990, p. 2)

These vignettes demonstrate how the interactions between caregiver and children can be distorted or short-circuited when parents respond out of their own needs or misread the signs and signals of their infants.

Movement therapy is a unique and integral part of the early intervention program at the facility in which this author (Blau) works. The facility is a day school for children 6 months to 10 years with developmental disabilities. Babies and their caregivers in the early intervention program come to school one or more times a week for therapeutic services that include speech, occupational, physical, and movement therapy. Children also receive educational services and parents participate in behavior management groups and group therapy. In the early intervention program, the caregiver and child are treated together with the focus on their relationship. Extensive evaluations and suggestions from staff and administration identify children whose social/emotional needs indicate that they would benefit from movement therapy. In addition to biweekly individual sessions, children are seen in group at least once a week. Relaxation techniques, rhythmic interactions, sensory awareness activities, and fine and gross motor play are some of the tools utilized to foster social/emotional growth by improving body image, self-esteem, and relatedness.

Early movement therapy intervention has shown itself to be successful in altering maladaptive patterns between infants and caregivers. The movement therapist, trained to observe changes in body movement including flow, shape, rhythm, and dynamics can utilize a nonverbal system of communication in order to bring about changes in unsuccessful patterns of interaction. Such a therapist is particularly able to help the parent translate nonverbal cues into meaningful child/parent "dialogues" and to sensitize the parent to the impact that a nonverbal system of communication has on a baby.

As stated above, at the facility, infants, ages 6 months to 2 $^1/_2$ years, are seen, at least once a week. The therapy takes place in a carpeted therapy room about 6' x 10' with a floor mat and one-way mirror. Equipment includes a bean bag, pillows, blankets, a standing mirror, phonograph and records, Nerf™ balls, lotion, a child's-size table, two child-size chairs, and an adult-size rocking chair. The baby and primary caregiver are treated together; other family members are included when appropriate. Sessions emphasize the family context of infant development and the need to foster a child's growth as a person, no matter how severe the impairment.

Although, initially, the caregiver may view the baby as the client, ultimately the caregiver learns the importance of treating the relationship and, in this context, all family members are seen as clients. The transition from seeing the baby as the client to seeing the family as the client is often met with defensiveness and resistance. It takes the careful and skillful building of an alliance between the therapist and caregiver to achieve this goal. As the caregiver feels vulnerable concerning her own mothering skills, the therapist must be seen as understanding, noncritical, and supportive. The therapist must support the caregiver's strengths as a mother and be sure to focus on these strengths. When addressing weaknesses, the therapist needs to approach the parent in a gentle manner and make suggestions rather than critical statements. A period of time during which the therapist joins with the caregiver by merely observing her with her baby and engaging in general conversation should precede any interventions or feedback. This helps the caregiver feel comfortable and allied with the therapist.

Movement sessions focus on the spontaneous interactions that occur between parent and child and the material for intervention lies in what is happening between the baby and parent at any particular moment. It is important that during a session, the parent and child are given an opportunity to "be together" without focusing on "fixing" the handicap. For example:

Mark, a 10 month old, has cerebral palsy and is unable to control the movements of his limbs. The therapist encourages his mother to observe Mark's facial movements. Mark is wriggling his nose and sticks out his tongue. His mom is encouraged to respond to these movements by copying them and tuning into their rhythmic pattern so that a turn-taking interaction takes place. Mark looks surprised and pleased that his mother has affirmed his activity. Mother and baby engage in a nose-wriggling, tongue-wagging dialogue that brings smiles and laughter. (Debi Karlinksy, personal communication, 1994)

In this interaction, the parent became aware that her baby could "reach out" in unusual ways. Focusing on what the infant could do was a relief from endless hours spent on improving his disabilities (i.e., following numerous exercises aimed at building strength and coordination). In contrast, movement therapy treatment was aimed at enhancing sensorimotor capacities rather than alleviating deficits. The therapist helped the caregiver make use of her infant's existing strengths to make meaningful contact with the environment.

Another general goal of sessions is to encourage caregivers to relinquish control of their infant's behavior in favor of attending to the baby's spontaneous activities. Sessions focus on support of infant-initiated activities in order to facilitate changes in child/caregiver interactions. Spontaneous cues are built into playful interactions that are appropriate for the child's level of development.

The following are examples of parents' supporting child-initiated behavior:

Jenny, a 10 month old, becomes excited over a new toy. She reaches for it while exclaiming a joyful "oooh." She looks at her mother who returns her gaze while raising her shoulders and quickly shaking her head back and forth. Mother's response is excited, joyful and lasts as long as Jenny's. (Stern, 1985, p. 140)

Andy, a 9 month old, extends his arm, stretches his fingers and leans towards a toy in an effort to reach it. He still can't quite touch it. Andy tenses his body and stretches further. At that moment, his father wrinkles his nose, tenses his vocal cords and expels the sound "ugh...ugh" matching his son's effort to reach the toy. Dad's vocal effort and expression reflect his baby's physical behavior. (Stern, 1985, p. 140)

By synchronizing their responses, these parents teach their babies that experiences can be shared. By modifying the level and intensity of their reactions in response to the child's, these caregivers match the children's spontaneous behaviors and, thus, insure the increased attention and mutual attunement necessary for secure attachment (Stern, 1985).

Of course harmonious interactions positively influence growth but a perfect "fit" is not always necessary or even optimal. Babies' needs change from moment to moment. Parents and children constantly adjust their behaviors to each other and provide varying levels and types of stimulation.

There is an optimal interaction level during which time parents provide children with just the right amount and type of stimulation wanted and needed. But, there are times when caregivers provide more stimulation than the infant can handle or not enough stimulation and restlessness occurs. Sometimes, parents may ignore children's signals. All these parental responses teach the baby that not all experiences can be shared and this, in turn, lays the groundwork for separation from the mother/infant bond.

For healthy development to take place, all young children need to experience interactions that promote attachment and interactions that promote separateness (Mahler, 1970). In a well-functioning system, children need to be both attached and separate. It is when the caregiver is not tuned into the babies' needs or when there are incongruent behaviors (behaviors that send contradictory messages) that a dysfunctional relationship can occur.

There are a number of behaviors that promote attachment. Prolonged gazing into each other's eyes is always significant. Sharing a focus is more complex and can involve an object, event, or feeling that affects both partners rather than meeting the exclusive needs of one. For example, a mother and child sway together while listening to a musical selection. Movement that results in physical contact and molding is even more subtle. Molding occurs when two people accomodate their body shapes and rhythmic patterns to each other. For example, during nursing a mother creates a "cradle," with her arm and upper torso, into which her baby can "snuggle" while she strokes or taps her infant's body in rhythm to his sucking. Behaviors that promote separateness include exploration of objects in the external world, bodily resistance to the shape and rhythms of the partner, nonverbal cues that communicate needs, dislikes, or wishes as opposed to the passive acceptance of the adult's suggestions (Dulicai & Silberstein, 1984).

Dulicai and Silberstein (1984) describe a wide category of incongruent behaviors that promote dysfunction. These behaviors encompass any activity containing contradictory messages. For example,

> A mother may offer a child a puzzle to play with. She displays it for examination with quickness and strength while at the same time maintaining a tight grasp that prevents the child from accepting it; the message "this is for you" is contradicted by "you can't take this from me." (pp. 64-65)

During movement-therapy sessions, therapists help parents become aware of their infant's spontaneous communications. The parents are helped to focus on the nonverbal parameters needed in order to develop synchronous patterns of interaction. Nonverbal behaviors that are observed include: (a) the infant's and parent's use of personal space (the space that can be reached by extending one's arms): do the mother and baby share the same personal space or is there a distance maintained? (b) direction of gaze: do the baby and mother gaze into each other's eyes? Do they maintain a shared focus or do they pay attention to different things? (c) body attitude: are their bodies relaxed and open or constricted and tense? Does the mother hover? (d) molding: do mother and baby appear comfortable when in close physical contact? Does the mother respond to her baby's need to readjust his body? (e) exploratory/blocking behavior: does mother facilitate or interfere with her child's attempts to explore the environment? (f) contact seeking/avoiding patterns: do mother and infant seek contact or do they avoid each other? Is contact maintained through eye gaze or voice while child and caregiver are at a distance? (g) rhythmic interaction: do the rhythmic patterns of mother's movements, breath, and voice clash with or complement her baby's? and (h) the degree of match or mismatch of movement qualities: are both partners moving with a similar intensity or is one quick while the other is slow, perhaps even lethargic and passive?

The following are brief examples of the ways in which movement interventions can influence dysfunctional parent/child relationships:

> Pat and her 4-month-old baby, Tom, are seated on a straight-back chair. Pat is holding her baby ventrally, in the crook of her arm, while vigorously rocking him. Her torso is stiff and her respiration is shallow and arrhythmic. Tom is wriggling uncomfortably. His gaze is averted. The therapist suggests that Pat and Tom move to a comfortable rocking chair and that Pat cradle Tom in the crook of her knee and simultaneously stroke his body. She is encouraged to breathe deeply, relax her torso and rock gently and rhythmically to a quiet, musical selection. Tom's body relaxes as he molds into the space created by Pat's bent knee. Pat looks down at her baby and eye contact is made. Tom reaches for his mother's face. (Blau, 1989, p. 2)

Initially, the mother does not respond to her child's nonverbal cues. The infant averts his gaze and wriggles with discomfort as the mother rocks him. Her body posture and rhythmic pattern attest to her nervousness. They move to a rocking chair; deep breathing while listening to quiet music allows the mother to slow down. The therapist has enabled the mother to become consciously aware of her own body rhythms and the need to quiet them in order to calm her baby. Responding to the possibility that the baby may need greater distance, the mother is encouraged to hold him further away. The infant responds by molding, gazing into his mother's eyes, and reaching out for additional contact.

In the following, a miscommunication occurs when the parent "reads" the baby's mind instead of attending to his nonverbal signals.

Jane and her 10 month old, Paul, are seated on the floor. Jane is disappointed in play with her son because of his lack of response. Paul crawls behind a standing mirror in the therapy room. Jane interprets his act as Paul's wish to avoid interaction with her. The therapist suggests that Jane follow her son's lead by moving to the mirror and engaging him in a peek-a-boo game, using the mirror as a barrier. Baby and mother tentatively begin the peek-a-boo but Jane lacks affective involvement and the volume of her voice is too low. The therapist suggests that she speak louder and concentrate on matching her voice and affect to the excitement inherent in the game of peek-a-boo. Jane experiments with changing her affect and voice volume until her behavior is in the range of tolerance and stimulation which attracts her son's attention. To her delight, he greets her with a big smile and the play develops into a rhythmic dance which is fulfilling to both mother and child. (Blau, 1989, pp. 2–3)

In this intervention, the therapist has altered what would have become a negative interaction. The mother is able to observe that if she follows her son's lead, she can engage him. She learns what Murphy (1979) points out: if her invitation to play is "too weak, the baby rejects it, whereas if the level of intensity, feeling and movement is within the range of the baby's interest and tolerance, the baby is more apt to respond positively" (p. 63). The mother becomes sensitized to the need to modify her level of affect in response to her child's feedback.

These examples indicate that observations of nonverbal relationship patterns are a clue to effective strategies; that parents can be made aware of the need to accommodate their own nonverbal behaviors to foster their child's growth.

Early intervention designed to remediate relationship patterns, such as those described, is necessary to lay the groundwork for optimal development. Although early intervention programs have not yet been mandated as an educational service, it is clear that early intervention for vulnerable infants and their families is vital for the prevention and remediation of developmental disabilities.

14

Treating Children with Autism in a Public School System

Tina Erfer

What is it like to be in a room with six autistic children? Sometimes it is as if you are among six distinct planets in a strange solar system, while still within the same four walls. Sometimes it may feel lonely, as though you are the only one in the room. But, if you enter with a spirit of openness and acceptance, you also experience the joy and fascination of being with some very special children.

Who are these children? What are they like? What might it feel like to be autistic? And what does dance/movement therapy offer children with autism?

The intent of this chapter is to review theoretical material regarding diagnosis and etiology of autism, to discuss the rationale for using dance/movement therapy with groups of children so diagnosed, and to illustrate goals and methodology through specific examples of group sessions.

Diagnosis

Autism is not a disease. It is a behaviorally defined developmental disability that affects sociability, language, and a variety of brain functions.

It has been said that whether or not a child is diagnosed as autistic depends on who makes the diagnosis. Much controversy has centered around autism, from diagnosis to etiology (Victor, 1983; Wing, 1976). The clinical observations made by Kanner in 1943, however still form the basis for subsequent theories about the condition. Kanner (1955) writes that:

> The common denominator in all these patients is a disability to relate themselves in the ordinary way to people and situations from the beginning of life....The case histories indicate...the presence from the start of autistic aloneness which...shuts out anything that comes to the child from the outside. (p. 717)

A number of other characteristics are described by Kanner (1955) and other researchers (Bettelheim, 1967; Ruttenberg, Kalish, Wenar, Wolf, 1977; Wing, 1976). Some infants evidence autistic symptoms such as failing "to assume the usual anticipatory posture prepatory to being picked up" (Kanner, 1955, p. 717). Other children develop normally and then after 15 to 20 months, there is a regression that "involves withdrawal from physical and emotional contact with people" (Ruttenberg, et al., 1977, p. 6).

Many children diagnosed as autistic exhibit self-stimulating and perseverative behaviors, such as hand-flapping and rocking; even head-banging and other forms of self-injury are seen. Such children have a tendency to handle toys and other objects primarily for sensory stimulation rather than for purposes of mastery or imaginative play. These children are often extremely active; they may move either in an unfocused and disorganized manner or in an obsessively repeated pattern through space. At the opposite extreme, other children are listless and passive, hardly moving at all unless prodded by an adult.

In addition to self-stimulating behaviors, problems of motor control are prevalent among children who are autistic. They may grimace or jump up and down when they are excited. They may rock from back foot to front foot, bending at the waist, while listening to music. When quiet, some have an awkward posture, head bowed, arms flexed at the elbow, hands drooping at the wrist. Many are toe-walkers, seeming unable to put the whole foot down. Some children show no signs of dizziness after prolonged spinning. Others have marked problems in motor imitation—the ability to learn by watching and imitating. This is particularly evident when movements have to be reversed in direction, as when a child waves his hand toward himself when saying goodbye. It is often possible for such children to learn motions if their limbs are moved for them. In addition, concepts such as left/right, up/down, and back/front may be confused.

In many cases there is a seeming lack of interest in or understanding of speech and language. "If speech is present, it is usually imitative, echolalic, and serves...a discharge function" (Ruttenberg, et al., 1977, p. 7). Such speech is marked by incorrect use of pronouns, pronomial reversal, and lack of the use of "I," as when the child uses "he," "she," "you," or the child's own name, instead of "I," when referring to him or herself.

Echolalia is the production of words or phrases that seem to be an exact copy of those originally spoken by another person. Echolalic speech can be immediate or delayed and often seems irrelevant to the current activity or situation. Sometimes echoed phrases are stored and later used in their entirety when a particular stimulus occurs. For example, a child might say "put the ball in the box" rather than a more appropriate greeting when he or she sees the movement therapist.

Among children designated as autistic there are often abnormal sensory responses that seem to derive from difficulty in making use of incoming information from all the senses. For example, a child may show no reaction to a sudden loud noise but may be oversensitive to a quiet, ordinary sound, such as a radiator hiss. Some children have abnormalities in their visual inspection behavior, using peripheral rather than central vision. There may be apparent difficulty in recognizing things or people, an inability to attend to that which is close while concentrating on a small detail at a distance. Poor eye contact and even active visual avoidance may be observed. These children are often fascinated by lights, shiny objects, or particular patterns. Some children seem to be indifferent to pain or cold, but may display exaggerated concern with minor discomforts. These children seem to lack fear or awareness of real danger; at the same time, they may react with terror to apparently harmless situations. Some children are tactile-defensive, unable to tolerate touch. Others react with intense pleasure to particular tactile sensations, such as smooth surfaces, or may touch and stroke various textures obsessively. The same kinds of patterns may be observed with taste and smell.

There is often a tendency for such children to pay attention to only one aspect of a person, object, or scene, instead of the whole. There may seem to be a lack of response especially to other children, even if the ability to relate to adults improves. There is generally little understanding of other people's feelings. Laughing, giggling, crying, or screaming may occur for no apparent reason.

In many there is unpredictable and intense resistance to change, and an attachment to routines. "Reaction to change…is usually rage, panic or withdrawal" (Ruttenberg, et al., 1977, p. 7). At such times there is often a return to self-stimulating, perseverative behaviors.

Wing (1976) delineates several areas in which the "classically" autistic child may perform well despite his or her many impairments. These usually involve nonlanguage-dependent skills and skills that rely on exact memory. For example, a child may be adept at dismantling and assembling mechanical or electrical apparatus, puzzles, or toys. Some children show a marked love of music and a surprising ability to sing well. Others have the ability to store items in memory for prolonged periods of time in the exact form in which they were first experienced, as in echolalia. Such items seem to be stored, however, without being interpreted or changed. Some children remember the words of songs, lists of names, advertisements, conversations overheard, bus and train routes, or numerical calculations. But these items of memory cannot be applied appropriately to reality situations.

Because skills and abilities can co-exist with gross impairments, a general level of intelligence cannot be predicted from a special ability. In general, the autistic pattern of behavior can be associated with mental retardation of varying degrees of severity, with average intelligence, or even, in rare cases, with above-average intelligence.

Victor (1983) views autism as more than a set of symptoms and believes it is better described by the term "pervasive developmental disorder," as it seems to be a general adaptation or personality organization that affects all major aspects of life. Victor's term is the one used in the *Diagnostic and Statistical Manual of Mental Disorders* (DSM III-R), in which the "Autistic Disorder" is defined as having the essential features that constitute "a severe form of Pervasive Developmental Disorder, with onset in infancy or childhood" (APA, 1987, p.38). The features detailed in the DSM III-R are the same as those described previously. The diagnostic criteria in the DSM III-R must include at least 8 of 16 basic items listed and a criterion is considered to have been met only if the behavior is abnormal for the person's developmental level. Currently, educational evaluators and school psychologists frequently assign the diagnosis of pervasive developmental disorder (PDD) to children who exhibit many of the aforementioned criteria.

Etiology of Autism and Idiosyncratic Behaviors

Over the years, there has been much controversy regarding the etiology of autism (Bettleheim, 1967; Victor, 1983; Wing, 1976). Current research, however, seems to point to organic factors. Clinical observations and studies have led researchers to believe that some form of organic brain damage, biochemical imbalance, or disorder of brain development plays a major role in autism and related disorders of communication (Mnukhin & Isaev, 1975; Schmeck, 1988).

Based on his research, Courchesne (as cited in Schmeck, 1988) suggests that the autistic person may have a fragmentary view of life and that his or her "excessively stimulated brain is bombarded by confusing messages that only occasionally resolve into sensible patterns that can contribute to useful memory and development of personality"(p. c3). He postulates that autistic persons are born with brains that are abnormally subject to stimulation and that from early life such people try to shield themselves from extra stimulation. In his theory, "the autistic person's tendency to stare at blinking lights or spinning wheels is a way of coping with too much stimulation. There is a brain mechanism...through which such rhythmical experiences can have a calming effect on the activity of the cerebral cortex" (Courchesne as cited in Schmeck, 1988, p. c3).

It is important to remember that few generalizations regarding autistic children are ever completely accurate. Children with autistic behavior may appear to be at any point on a range from seeming to need to block out perceived sensory overload to seeming to crave more and more stimulation. Benbow (1977) views the behavior rituals of children who appear to crave stimulation as attempts to satisfy specific, basic sensory needs. Rocking and whirling respond to the need for vestibular and kinesthetic stimulation, which relates to body movement, weight, and position in space. Jumping and darting are in response to the need for proprioceptive input, and a variety of skin receptor stimulations seem to satisfy tactile needs. Benbow considers these rituals the autistic person's attempt to "self-treat" using specific areas in which the greatest number of tactile receptors are located, the mouth, the palms of hands, and the soles of the feet. In addition, some self-injurious or self-mutilating behaviors are thought to occur as a result of a heightened sensory threshold within the brain stem. "The longer the child 'treats' a specific area, the more drastic (even to the point of destruction of tissue) the stimulus will need to become to be appreciated by the child" (Benbow, 1977, p. 46). In addition, the longer the ritual has been carried on, the harder it is to eliminate.

The neural development of children with autism is so irregular, and fluctuates so widely without apparent external cause, that Benbow (1977) calls autistic children "sensory puzzles" (p. 43). If, for example, an autistic child withdraws from group play, it is difficult to determine whether the withdrawal is due to tactile defensiveness, such as aversion to touch; due to postural insecurity, which is an inability to maintain balance while moving or a fear of movement through space; due to vestibular dysfunction; to a combination of these; or due to social–emotional factors.

Victor (1983) puts forth the hypothesis that "autistic children are born with defective communication systems and, therefore, fail to provide cues for maternal behavior. Consequently, their mothers do not provide care that infants require for normal development" (p. 83). Therefore, even if the etiology involves an organic "first cause," the course of autistic development will probably still be "psychological insofar as experiences critical in autism are tied to the interaction of infant and caretaker" (Victor, 1983, p. 246). Thus, there is a connection between the caretaker's patterns of holding and carrying the infant and early vestibular and tactile stimulation. In turn this interrelationship greatly influences the development of body image, which will be discussed later in this chapter.

Wing (1976) also views autistic children as extremely vulnerable to environmental pressures. Problems arise particularly because they need highly specialized methods of child rearing in order for them to compensate for their specific impairments. It is common to find that when parents attempt to bring up their autistic child in "the normal way," the child then develops a series of secondary behavior problems,

> because he is not normal and is confused by the talk, social interaction, and general give-and-take of normal family life. The parents, in turn, also react with confusion because of the strange behavior of their child. They veer between over-permissiveness and inappropriate attempts to impose control. It is only when and if the parents learn, through professional help, or more often, through trial and error, the special techniques that are necesary, that the problems can be alleviated. (p. 80)

Unfortunately, there are parents or caretakers who themselves have abnormal or problematic personalities, and there are parents who find they cannot come to terms with such a difficult child. For example, cases of parental substance abuse, of course, not only have a profound effect on prenatal development resulting in neurological impairment or brain damage, but such parents are unable to provide the most basic childcare.

The interplay between organic and psychological factors is well-established. Therefore, therapy for autism must address the neurological or physical impairments in conjunction with the social/emotional disabilities. Careful study of the children's experience is essential to the understanding of their behavior, and to the development of preventive and remedial programs.

Rationale for the Use of Dance/Movement Therapy

Dance/movement therapy is ideally suited for working with the autistic population. Movement is a universal means of communication. All children move in some way, and those who are autistic are no exception. Because the autistic child usually has not developed communicative speech, but has a unique movement "language," nonverbal communication is an effective means of contact.

"Few experiences involve the total person as completely as that of dance action: the body, the emotions, and the mind. Moving with other people in a similar rhythm often helps relationships to form" (Chace,1957, as cited in Sandel, Chaiklin, and Lohn, 1993, pp. 343–44). Communication through movement helps a child to be more aware of him- or herself and more able to interact with others. Through various techniques that will soon be discussed, the dance therapist works toward the development of trust and the formation of a relationship.

Leventhal (1981) states that dance/movement therapy for the special child "deals fundamentally with sensory motor and perceptual motor development and integration; ultimately building the body image and developing the self-concept" (p. 1). Sensorimotor activities combine full-body movement and the sensory input that such movement provides. Perception refers to the meaning the brain gives to sensory input, through the process of organizing or interpreting the raw data obtained through the senses. Perceptual–motor integration involves the interaction of the various channels of perception, visual, auditory, tactile, and kinesthetic, with motor activity.

Body image is one of the most fundamental concepts in human growth and development and one that appears to be lacking in children who are autistic. Schilder (1950) defines body image as the three-dimensional picture or image of our own body that we form in our mind, the way in which the body appears to ourselves. Without a body image, a symbol of one's own body,

> the psychic structures necessary for symbolic representation of other things cannot be formed, since they depend on previous symbolization. Consequently,...the autistic child develops no words to form ideas; he cannot make the bridge from the concrete to the abstract;...and...is functionally unaware of object, self, or world. (Dratman & Kalish, 1967, p. 7)

Body image has a physiological basis. It is based on input from the vestibular, kinesthetic, proprioceptive, tactile, and visual systems. The development of body image parallels sensorimotor development. This, in turn, forms the basis for the sense of self, cognitive development, the acquisition of self-help skills, and for many basic concepts.

Schilder (1950) highlights the correlation between movement and the body image. He states that "movement leads to a better orientation in relation to our own body....We do not know very much about our body unless we move it....[and] movement is a great uniting factor between the different parts of our body" (p. 112). He goes on to say that in order to build a body image we have to know where our limbs are, and we must also be aware of the relationship of the different body parts to each other. Schilder states that movement experiences can lead from a change in body image to a change in the psyche.

Many dance/movement therapists agree with Schilder (1950) that "by movement we come into a definite relation to the outside world and to objects.... [and,]...only by movement and new contacts with the outside world will the knowledge about our own body increase" (pp. 113–114). Chace (1964, as cited in Sandel, Chaiklin, & Lohn, 1993) writes that dance therapy, "in making use of the basic form of communication, offers the individual a means of relating himself to the environment or to people when he is cut off...by the patterns of his illness" (p. 245).

The more defined one's body image, the better one is able to differentiate oneself from the environment and from others. This differentiation is necessary for the formation of relationships. Therefore, movement and the body image are two of the dance/movement therapist's major concerns when addressing the needs of children with autism.

A guiding principle for dance/movement therapy with autistic children is the synthesis of the physical and relational aspects of the work. No matter what physical skill or ability is in focus, the fundamental, and often primary, emphasis is on developing a relationship between human beings. Behavioral change occurs through, and is supported by, the interpersonal relationship established with the child (or children) through movement. Significant changes that occur on the movement level can affect total functioning (Schmais, 1974). Therefore, by broadening or expanding a child's movement repertoire, we provide him or her with a wider range of skills to use in understanding and coping with the environment. It is important to note that this work is process-oriented, rather than product-oriented.

It can't be emphasized enough how important the awareness of his or her physical self is to a child's ability to organize impulses and internalize controls. Children must understand their own bodies and their capacity for movement before they can cope with the external demands of the environment. In other words, unless there is a sense of oneself as a separate entity, differentiated from others, one cannot effectively, or "affectively," relate beyond oneself.

The initial goals of dance/movement therapy are to reach the child at the level at which he or she seems to be functioning—the sensorimotor level, to establish a relationship, and to work toward the formation of a body image. These goals are concurrent and ongoing, woven into the fabric of the interactions between therapist and child.

Mirroring, a form of reflecting back but not imitating another's movements, provides a powerful means to understand a child's experience, on a body level. Not only does it give the therapist valuable information about a child that might not be discovered otherwise, but it also conveys to the child the message that she is being seen and accepted as she is. Such acceptance often causes a child to shift his or her focus from inner stimuli to stimuli in the environment, which then leads to increased connectedness and paves the way for reciprocal interactions. The therapist does not mirror a child who is out of control, or when the action does not seem to offer the possibility for a positive change in either the relationship or movement patterns. If a child has lost a sense of boundaries and safety, the therapist's job is not to reflect back but to provide structure, boundaries, and a sense of safety for the child. As the therapist gets to know the children, she or he will be able to detect the beginning of agitation and can structure the session (or a particular child's participation in the session) in such a way as to avoid loss of control. The therapist constantly monitors the mood, tone, and energy level of the group in order to assess when to change or modify activities or movement interventions. It is possible to use mirroring in a group context, for example, when the therapist chooses a particular song, activity, or prop that reflects the demonstrated energy or movement dynamics present in the group.

The dance/movement therapist always seeks to provide a consistent and accepting atmosphere, while working toward establishing a relationship with the autistic child. Often, this is a slow process that occurs on the child's terms. In addition to mirroring, the use of eye contact, touch, vocalization, rhythmic body action, music, various props, and a variety of sensorimotor activities all contribute to the building of a relationship, as well as to the development of body image.

Dance/movement therapy with groups of these children includes activities or interventions that involve basic sensory awareness, body-parts awareness, movement dynamics, locomotor movement and, eventually, more expressive movement. It is by means of experiences such as these, as well as tactile stimulation, identification of body parts and boundaries, and visual–kinesthetic awareness development, which is strenghthened by having children alternate between moving and observing others move, that children with autism may begin to develop self-and body-awareness.

A process called "sensory integration" provides additional opportunities for growth in the area of body–image formation. Sensory integrative therapy includes full-body movements that provide vestibular, proprioceptive, and tactile stimulation, offering pleasurable sensory experiences to otherwise overstimulated or isolated children. The goal is to improve the way the brain processes and organizes sensations, so that the various parts of the nervous system work together to enable a person to interact with the environment effectively and experience appropriate satisfaction. Like dance/movement therapy, sensory integration therapy starts at the child's current level of functioning. It is based on the theory that a child cannot progress to a higher or more complex level of functioning until the prerequisite skills at the preceding level have developed. In order for a child to move beyond the sensorimotor stage of development, enough sensory integration has to take place to allow for the formation of adaptive responses. An adaptive response is a purposeful, goal-directed response to sensory experience, in which one masters a challenge and learns something new. This, in turn, helps the brain to develop and organize itself, ideally in an ongoing process. The combination of sensory integrative therapy and dance/movement therapy provides an interactive, supportive, and effective treatment approach for children who are autistic. This approach will be described more specifically in the following sections.

Structure of a Session

How an actual dance/movement therapy session is run is likely to vary, depending on the orientation and personality of the therapist, the nature of the facility, the functioning level of the children, and the goals and needs of both the setting and the children. There is a framework or basic structure inherent in all groups, however. Within this structure, the dance/movement therapist constantly addresses individual goals, while fostering group awareness and interaction through movement.

The session begins with a warm-up, which, in time, becomes an opening ritual, something familiar and secure that the children anticipate, and something that sets this time apart from the rest of the day. The warm-up is both an emotional and a physical preparation for what is to follow. It varies in length and type of movements, depending on the level of functioning, energy, and awareness of the group members. The present physical, psychological, and emotional states of the children when they enter the room is always taken into account and used as a starting point.

During the warm-up, the children are usually seated in chairs arranged in a circle, a formation that delineates the boundaries of the group and provides spatial organization and a center of focus. The chairs are used because it is often difficult for the children to remain focused while sitting on the floor or standing. Eye contact and recognition of each individual in the group is encouraged during the warm-up, as well as a sense of group awareness and cohesiveness.

The development of body image and body/self awareness is enhanced through isolation and identification of body parts. Naming body parts as they are touched and moved provides a cognitive link to the physical actions. Integration of body parts to whole-body awareness is developed through rhythmic movement—by bending, stretching, swaying, swinging, shaking, and stamping. Rhythm is a meaningful organizer of impulses, and singing the actions as they are performed establishes a rhythm for the group. Singing also promotes language development, communication, and expression. Group members are encouraged to try to sing to the best of their ability.

The therapist always supports the group's movements and sounds with verbalizations that describe everything being done by the group. During transitions the group is told in simple, concrete words that one activity is finished, and explains what the next activity will be. Combining the spoken word with gesture and movement aids in improving cognitive awareness of the actions. In addition, throughout the session, the therapist and adult assistants provide verbal and physical guidance to children who need additional support in order to participate.

The group progresses from moving body parts while seated to moving the entire body in a contained space to moving through space in the room. It is helpful if props and materials are kept out of sight until ready for use.

As the session progresses, a higher energy level is often reached. This part of the session, the development, is a time for working on concepts, developing themes, teaching and practicing motor skills, and developing socialization skills. Opportunities for large group movement activities alternate with interaction in dyads or small groups, individual movement exploration and one-to-one interactions with the therapist. In addition, vigorous activities always alternate with calmer, lower-energy activities in order to prevent overstimulation.

The closure of the session brings everyone back to the circle of chairs. It is a time for calming and centering the children, and for singing a "good-bye" song, which repeats the format of the "hello" song. It is also a transition that helps the children to return to their classroom with a sense of completion and accomplishment.

Music and props are two important elements in a group session. It is important to use music with a simple rhythmic structure as more complex rhythms may confuse an already fragmented or disorganized child. However, serene or meditative-type music may promote a mood of quiet at the end of the session or whenever deemed appropriate by the therapist.

Because props are concrete and external, they can serve to focus a child's or the group's attention. A prop, used as a bridge between therapist and child, enables the child to tolerate a relationship that might be too threatening if carried on more directly. A prop placed strategically in the center of a group not only focuses the attention of all the children, it also facilitates synchronous group movement. In sum, props have broader and more far-reaching positive effects than just their obvious use; they involve the social, emotional, cognitive, as well as physical realms.

Session structure provides the children a sense of having experienced something "whole"—with a clear beginning, middle, and end. When the structure is predictable and secure, the children feel safe enough to begin to take more risks in movement exploration and growth. Furthermore, the use of such a reliable and repeated structure facilitates the development of trust in the relationship between children and therapist.

It is important to emphasize that although groups of children are being discussed, each child is unique and individual goals are constantly being addressed within the context of the group. There are goals, however, which are common to many of these children and these goals are woven through the warm-up, development, and closure. All of the techniques described are applicable not only to children with autism but also to children with other disorders such as attention deficit, and brain damage.

Two Sessions

The following session descriptions illustrate the goals and methods outlined above. The first session is an example of a group of more severely impaired children than those in the second session. Most of the movement interventions and activities described, however, can be used with children on all levels of functioning, with modifications as appropriate.

Session One

The group is made up of four boys and one girl, ranging in age from 5 to 7. At the time this session took place, Luis, Rosa, and Raymond had been working with me for approximately 2 years; Peter and Jimmy had only recently joined the group.

Before the session began, the circle of chairs had been deliberately placed in a corner of the room so that two walls provided additional boundaries, as the children in this group have particular difficulty focusing. It is not easy for them to sit still, and they tend to move in quick disorganized patterns all around the room when in unstructured situations or open space. When the five children and the educational assistant entered the movement room I met them at the door and helped direct the children to the chairs. Luis and Raymond allowed me to hold their hands and walk with them, whereas the other two boys ran in opposite directions into the room. Rosa stood by the door for a few minutes, and then slowly tip-toed to a chair and sat down. Once all the children were gathered together in the circle of chairs, the assistant and I positioned ourselves next to the children who needed the most direct support and guidance in order to participate.

When everyone was seated, I counted out loud to three as a signal that we were about to begin our usual opening song and then all of us sang "Now it's time for movement...," a song with a very simple rhythmic beat. When we finished, I handed a puppet to Peter, who was sitting next to me, to begin the "Hello" song. Everyone now sang "hello" to him, and he was encouraged to move the puppet in the same rhythm as the song. When Peter's turn was finished he was told to look at Rosa, who was sitting next to him, and to pass the puppet to her. We all continued until everyone had a turn, including the adults.

After the "hello" song, the puppet was put away, and a Nerf™ ball brought out. I demonstrated and verbally described what was to be done next. Then each person had a turn to hold the ball, place it on his or her head, squeeze it, and then pass it to the next person. The foam ball was, in turn, squeezed on heads, shoulders, arms, stomachs, backs, legs, and feet, while each body part was named as it was touched with the ball. Again, the students were encouraged to verbalize what they were doing, and were reminded to look at the person to whom they were passing the ball. Help was given, as needed, both physically and verbally, throughout the session, in order to promote success. For example, Jimmy threw the ball to the other side of the room, at first, and needed hand-over-hand assistance with this activity. And Raymond had to be reminded several times to pass the ball to the next person, rather than keep it for himself. The Nerf™ ball was returned to its place after everyone had a turn.

Next, the "Big Blue Ball," a large therapy balance ball (sometimes called a physioball), was put in the center of the circle of chairs. We all moved our chairs close enough to the ball so that we could touch it with outstretched hands. With accompanying physical demonstration, I directed everyone in turn to place a different body part on the ball, while singing what was being done in a simple rhythmic melody. A wide range of movement dynamics was used. Hands tapped the ball in a moderate rhythm, arms and hands pushed the ball strongly, fingers quickly and lightly touched the ball, elbows leaned slowly, heads rested on the ball softly, feet kicked or pushed and then rested on top of the ball. Each of these actions was performed repeatedly, working toward group synchrony, before going on to the next action.

After this time of synchronous group movement, the circle was widened by pushing the chairs back, maintaining the circle in a larger form. Now, one at a time, the children were helped up onto the large therapy ball. They lay on their stomachs or their backs, while I gently placed my hands on their backs or shoulders to support them, and to help them feel safe. The touch was important in helping to define body boundaries, and in establishing a relationship with each child. The children were rocked foward and back or side to side on the ball, and this also was reinforced by singing about the actions. Rocking on the therapy ball can be a nurturing and pleasurable experience for a child, while also providing his or her system with vestibular and proprioceptive stimulation. As the children were comfortable with being on the ball, they were given the choice as to how they would like to be positioned while being rocked, on their stomachs, backs, or sitting up. I noticed that Rosa clung fearfully to me if I tried to encourage her to lie on her back on the ball, so I allowed her to remain sitting upright. I always remained aware of the children's reactions, and never forced a fearful or insecure child to participate. The children were encouraged to watch each other being rocked on the ball. Luis and Raymond even put their hands on the ball while each of their classmates were sitting on it, and helped rock them from side to side.

After each of the children had several turns, I detected that their attention span was diminishing, so I announced that "the big blue ball is finished." The ball was now returned to its storage place and the chairs were moved to the side of the room against a wall, where the children again sat down.

It was now time for individual movement exploration. I brought out a variety of props, and placed them around the room. These included large mats on the floor, a tunnel to crawl through, two playground balls, two scooters, two hoops, several large geometric shapes (made of vinyl-coated foam) to climb on, and a few pieces of fabric of varying sizes. The children were invited to get up from their chairs, and choose whichever props they wanted to explore. The assistant and I moved through the room, interacting with the children, providing support, guidance, and encouragement. During this time, there were opportunities for brief one-to-one interactions with each of the children. Whenever possible, I engaged in mirroring the essence of each child's movement qualities and patterns.

Jimmy immediately ran to one of the playground balls, and sat on it, bouncing up and down. Peter was encouraged to join him, and sit on the other ball so they could bounce together. I brought over a large hoop for both of them to hold onto while they bounced as a way to foster interaction between them. The assistant helped Rosa and Luis as they climbed on the large foam shapes and rolled down the other side. Raymond seemed content to crawl into the tunnel and stay there. After bouncing with Jimmy and Peter for a while, I went over to Raymond in the tunnel. I sat at one end and watched and waited. A few minutes went by before he seemed to notice that I was there. I called his name, and commented that he was in the tunnel, while I was outside it. Slowly, he began to roll over first to one side, then to the other, causing the tunnel to roll away from where I was sitting and then toward me. I remained sitting where I was, but continued to describe what he was doing, and to remind him that I was still there. Eventually, the tunnel stopped moving and Raymond emerged. He then picked up a small ball and tossed it to me as if to say "let's play." After the individual movement exploration, it was "cleanup time," and I enlisted the help of the children to put all the props away. The children who were not yet able to do this were assisted in returning to the chairs to wait for the circle to be formed once again. When everyone was seated in the circle of chairs, we listened to quiet music, and began the closure of the session. The children were encouraged to take a deep breath after watching me demonstrate first, and finally they were asked to catch soap bubbles blown their way. Even the most unfocused child has been known to focus on a bubble, and try to catch it!

The session ended with a good-bye song. The puppet was brought out again. First, "this is the end of Movement" was sung by the whole group, and then each child was sung to in the same manner as in the warm-up. The children were then escorted out of the movement room, back to their classroom.

Session Two

The children in this group were functioning at a higher level that those in the first group, and had been working with me for 2 to 3 years. This group consisted of six boys, Don, Ramon, Tommy, Shawn, Matthew, and Alex, who were all 7 or 8 years old.

Because most of the boys in this group had been working longer than the first group, they were more familiar with established routines. They were also more able to communicate using verbal language, and often would remind me if I forgot to do something. For example, Shawn would always say "it's time for the purple ball" at the appropriate time. And Alex would become extremely agitated if we changed the order of the usual activities.

As I opened the door of the movement room, I was greeted with a burst of energy as the boys dashed straight to the circle of chairs in the corner of the room. They were ready to start, and could hardly wait for the adults to be seated.

This session began with the warm-up, as usual, with the group singing the opening songs. Since these boys were older we used a tambourine instead of a puppet, and encouraged the children to play the tambourine in the same rhythm as the songs.

After the "hello" song came a body awareness activity designed to warm up the children's muscles and begin to establish group synchrony. The activity was accompanied by recorded music that had a simple rhythmic beat but no lyrics. With demonstration and assistance, as needed, the children began to stretch up, reach down, stretch their arms foward toward the center of the circle, and bend down to touch and tap their own feet, their legs, knees, all the way up to shoulders and head. As the music continued, everyone then held hands in the circle, and sang words describing the actions as they swung their arms, shook hands, and moved arms up and down together. They also moved their bodies side to side and forward and back, swinging their legs, stamping and sliding their feet on the floor.

Then we stood up, still inside the circle of chairs, our movements were contained, but began to take up more space, and involve more whole-body actions. I offered: "stand up on your toes"; " bend down and be very small"; " lift your knees high and touch one at a time." When Shawn called out "stamp your feet," we joined him and stamped our feet. I asked the others for suggestions of what to do next, and Don began to spin around in a circle. I structured this into an action that could be done safely by everyone by saying "everyone turn around one time and stop!" The assistant and I made sure the children all stopped after only one turn by reaching out to hold their hands again immediately.

After eliciting at least one movement suggestion from each child, the group was led away from the chairs into the center of the room. A circle was reformed here, everyone holding hands again, and the group first walked and then skipped around in one direction and then the other. Then we moved into and out of the center, coming close and then moving apart. The music continued to accompany the action, providing a rhythmic organization to the session. As always, I constantly verbalized what was being done, and where and how it was being done.

At this point, I let go of one of Ramon's hands, instructing him and everyone else to continue holding on. The circle had now opened up to become a line, or a "train," weaving its way in a serpentine path around the room. As the first leader, I led the group in left turns and right turns around the room, always aware of each child's ability to follow and stay connected while holding hands and walking. Matthew let go a few times and we all paused while the assistant retrieved him from the other side of the room. Each person had a turn to be first, and to choose the direction in which the group traveled. Tommy began to walk in smaller and smaller circles when he was leading, and needed to be gently steered in a new direction with my hand holding his. After everyone had one turn to lead, various props were set up in a random arrangement in the room, as "obstacles" for the "train" to climb over, walk around, go through, slide under, walk and balance on, or step into. I continuously emphasized safety by reminding the children to look where they were going.

Although it was easier for some of the children than others to remain focused on this activity, their pleasure was evident. They often asked to do it in later sessions by requesting the particular music we usually used as accompaniment. After the "train" had run its course, and everyone had more than one chance to lead and follow, the children were asked to help put all the props away. A circle was formed once again, and while holding hands for support, the children were asked to experiment with balancing on one foot. I helped each child in the group to experience what it felt like to lift his leg higher off the ground, and at the same time physically supported him in his efforts. My goals at this point were to help the children develop or improve their balance, and to increase their focusing ability, impulse control, body awareness, and muscular strength. In addition, they also were learning how to work together, as they held each other's hands for support while balancing. After this, the group was asked to sit down, where they were, on the floor. They were directed to take deep breaths, and to do some simple stretches of the muscles and body parts that had been used during the session. I demonstrated and did the stretches along with the children.

The energy in the room was at a lower level now, and the children returned to their chairs, arranging them in a circle, for the closure. The music was now a slow, peaceful melody. A ball with a highly textured surface was passed around the circle. Each child was asked to hold the ball, feel its softness, and then give it to the next person. They were reminded to look at each other when passing the ball. This helped to calm and center the children, while offering an experience of sensory awareness and focusing, as well. Then the children were given a chance to take turns blowing soap bubbles for each other to catch. This was Tommy's favorite activity, and he stood in the center of the circle and blew bubbles to each of the others in turn. He made sure the adults had a turn as well. The session ended with the ending and good-bye songs, with bells, instead of the tambourine, to maintain the sense of quietness and calm that had developed.

Summary

The different functioning levels of the two groups of children is evident from the descriptions of the sessions. Each individual child had his or her own strengths and areas needing improvement, whereas each group as a whole developed a unique quality as well.

As the sessions illustrate, a dance/movement therapist working with groups of autistic children stresses the expansion of existing skills and cognitive abilities, while at the same time working toward the children's greater self-awareness, independence, and ability to relate to others. This is done through the use of touch, mirroring, games, rhythmic body actions, dance, music, and a variety of interactive experiences. Verbalizations are used to provide a concrete, cognitive link to the physical actions.

In groups, the choices of which movement intervention to use, and when, depend on the therapist's observations of nonverbal behaviors and attention to communication from individuals, and the overall tone of the group as a whole. The individual and group goals need to be blended into a meaningful experience for all.

In order for dance/movement therapists to effectively use their own bodies to interact with autistic children whose movement behaviors are often extreme and unusual, it is necessary for therapists to be especially familiar with their own movement repertoires. They need to observe the nonverbal communication from the children closely, to be constantly aware of their own nonverbal communication, and find ways for their own body movements to communicate with those of the children. By doing so the therapist can promote communication and interaction on a body level. Kalish (1968) describes this process as a delicate one. If the therapist intervenes too much, a child may withdraw; if there is not enough intervention, the child may not be reached at all. When working with groups, the need for this sensitivity is multiplied.

The intent of this work is always to involve children actively in a supportive environment that presents alternatives for their maladaptive functioning. Dance/movement therapists have a complex task—effecting changes in cognition, physical functioning, language development, feelings, and behavior.

Marian Chace emphasized the need for dance therapists to "have their 'antennae' attuned to their clients on all levels…and to sense, observe, respond, and act as catalyst to the client's potential selves as well as to their presented selves" (Downes, 1980, pp.14).

Implementation in the Public Schools

Many dance/movement therapists want to work with children in general and children with autism, in particular. In the current job market, opportunities to do so may often be found in the public school system. This is a viable option, as long as one is willing to understand the educational system and how dance/movement therapy fits into such a system. The political ramifications of this situation are beyond the scope of this chapter. The work can be and is being done to the benefit of the children involved, however.

In the New York City Public School System, the program that is called a "Specialized Instructional Environment" focuses on what the school system calls "Functional Life Skills with Communication Emphasis." It provides a highly structured environment designed to integrate instructional and supportive services throughout the school day; intensive speech and language training, and job-development services (for the older students) are provided. There is emphasis on the generalization of skills beyond the classroom, parent/guardian participation, and tasks taught and practiced in the home, school, and community. Four learning areas are emphasized: (a) social skills to help students relate to self, peers, family, school, and community; (b) communication skills for independent functioning; (c) personal self-help for independence in daily living; and (d) functional academic skills. Supportive services may include adaptive physical education, toilet training, travel training (for adolescent students), or occupational therapy. Everything is available to students if specified on their Individualized Education Program (IEP), which is written after a student is tested and evaluated by the Committee on Special Education.

There are two areas in which dance/movement therapists are commonly employed in the public school system—both within the Division of Special Education: as an Adaptive Physical Education teacher and in a "coverage" position. Adaptive Physical Education is defined (by the Regulations of the New York State Commissioner of Education) as a "...specially designed program of developmental activities, games, sports, and rhythms suited to the interests, capacities, and limitations of students with handicapping conditions who may not safely or successfully engage in unrestricted participation in the activities of the regular physical education program" (New York City, Public Schools—Division of Special Education, p. 20, 1991). In the New York City area, this service is mandated by the state for students who are autistic.

A "coverage" position involves relieving a classroom teacher from teaching responsibilities for a period, during which time a specified subject area is taught to the students. In programs for the autistic, these two positions are sometimes combined into one position, and it can be filled by a dance/movement therapist. Scheduling needs of a special education unit in a school generally dictate how many times per week each class is seen and whether or not there is time available for individual sessions in addition to the required groups.

Various areas of the country have different regulations governing special education programs and who may be hired to conduct these programs. There are states where dance/movement therapy is considered a "Related Service," similar to occupational and physical therapy, but, as of this writing, this is not the case in New York. In order for a dance/movement therapist to be hired by the public school system in this state, she or he needs to have state certification in special education or physical education, for an adaptive physical education job. A master's degree in dance/movement therapy can then fulfill the requirement for a master's degree that is "functionally related" to one's job. Sometimes, a dance/movement therapist who is also a social worker or school psychologist will be employed by the school system as well. Most often, it is the local public relations work by dance/movement therapists "on site" that informs principals and supervisors about dance/movement therapy, and its efficacy with special education students.

Conclusions

As in any bureaucratic system, a dance/movement therapist working in an educational setting may encounter frustrating politics and countless obstacles. The challenge is to maintain the integrity of the art and science of the field, so that dance/movement therapy remains a healing process for children with autism.

If the message of dance/movement therapy is to be recognized and heard, the message needs to be in a form and in language acceptable to educators. It is necessary, therefore, for a therapist to be able to "translate" dance/movement therapy theory, goals, and methodology into the language of the educational system. In order to understand that system, and how dance/movement therapy can fit in to it, it is helpful to take coursework in special education, in addition to the dance/movement therapy training.

One encounters special concerns in dealing with children who are autistic. A therapist may experience feelings of frustration, rage, or helplessness, because of constant exposure to what is perceived as rejection, or to aggressive behavior, or to a wish to "cure" autism without the ability to do so.

New therapists, especially, have unrealistic expectations as to the outcome of their work with these children. The painful reality of the situation may lead to reactions in the therapist that can negatively affect the therapy. For this reason, among others, it may be helpful for a dance/movement therapist who works with autistic children to be involved in professional supervision and/or personal therapy, in order to sort out their own strong reactions to the behaviors they may be encountering every day at work. By becoming aware of, and dealing with these reactions, a therapist can gain insight, become more empathetic and receptive and therefore able to make therapeutic choices that best meet the needs of the children.

Because work with these children is physically as well as emotionally demanding and exhausting, it is important for the dance/movement therapist to do personal work that helps redefine his or her own body boundaries, for example, by getting a massage. Relaxation and grounding experiences such as yoga, dance, and exercise classes, are extremely valuable. These are all recuperative and healing experiences for the therapist, helping him or her to maintain a strong sense of self.

In much of the literature on autistic children, it is written that they do not form relationships with others. If one approaches these children with an open mind and heart, however, one can see that they have their own ways of relating. Their ways of relating are so unconventional that anyone coming into contact with them will inevitably have many questions. "The children hold the answers, and one must accept their way to find those answers" (Erfer, Goldsand, & Weinstock, 1988, p. 104).

15

The Case of Warren: A KMP Approach to Autism

Susan Loman

The Kestenberg Movement Profile (KMP), a system of movement notation and analysis, is currently being used by dance/movement therapists to enhance their skills at observation, diagnosis, treatment planning, and intervention (Lewis, 1984, 1986, 1993; Lewis & Loman, 1990, 1992; Loman, 1991; Loman & Brandt, 1992; Merman, 1990). The process of learning the KMP provides therapists with information about their own movement preferences and how these preferences may affect the movement relationships that develop during the course of therapy. The KMP includes developmental and psychoanalytic theory (A. Freud, 1965; Kestenberg, 1975, 1985a; Mahler, Pine, & Bergman, 1975; Schilder, 1950) together with systems of movement analysis (Bartenieff & Lewis, 1980; Dell, 1970; Laban & Lawrence, 1947; Lamb, 1965). It can be interpreted psychodynamically or be used as a survey of movement qualities in both normal and pathological populations. Knowledge of the KMP system can inform the therapist about the range of movement qualities available to individuals of all ages.

The following case illustrates the use of the KMP therapy with an autistic child. Describing the sessions week by week preserves the sequential nature of the work and helps identify themes that pertain to specific phases in treatment. A clear progression from one phase to another is exemplified.

KMP Terminology

To aid the reader in understanding the terminology, KMP movement terms are bold-faced throughout the chapter and briefly defined in footnotes the first time they appear. These definitions are intended to clarify the text and do not include all of the terms contained in a complete KMP. Interested readers are referred to *The Role of Movement Patterns in Development, Volume II,* by Judith S. Kestenberg and K. Mark Sossin, for a full description of the Kestenberg Movement Profile System, including a glossary.

Oral Phase

Oral Sucking. During the first half year of life, an infant seeks union with primary caregivers through smooth rocking movements. These "sucking rhythms" originate in the mouth and serve the needs of sucking for nourishment as well as self-soothing. The rhythms spread throughout the body and serve the task of attachment. The primary plane in which movement takes place is the horizontal. Children in this phase enjoy putting objects in their mouths and sucking on them: pacifiers, fingers, toys, blankets all serve as pleasurable objects for this purpose.

Oral Biting. With the advent of teething in the second half of the first year, an infant begins to bite to alleviate oral discomfort. "Biting rhythms" are characterized by sharp transitions from contracted to released muscle tension. They serve the practical function of cutting through solid food as well as the developmental functions of separation and boundary formation. The child enjoys patting and tapping, shaking rattles, clapping games, and banging on any convenient surface.

Anal Phase

Anal Twisting. Beginning at the end of the first year and continuing into the beginning of the second year, the child becomes flexible at the waist and pelvis in the service of crawling and adjusting to spatial demands. "Anal twisting" rhythms appear in spinal motions that originate in the anal sphincter and spread throughout the body. The child is playful, teasing, and coy and begins to practice more locomotor skills. At times, the child enjoys smearing food and such creative messiness as finger painting.

Anal Straining. Typical of an 18-month-old child, tasks in this phase are: the beginnings of bowel control, climbing skills, autonomy, stability, organization, confrontation, verticality, intentionality, presentation of self, and the adaptive approach to the force of gravity. In this phase the child makes the transition into the vertical plane, becoming upright to face the world. Children enjoy making things with clay, throwing objects into containers, and asserting themselves by saying "no" with great intensity. This is also the age of the start of temper tantrums.

Urethral Phase

Urethral Running. This developmental stage begins in the third year of life. Tasks are to master locomotion, carry out operations, and to learn to run although without yet being able to stop. It is a phase of free-flowing mobility and wandering with no specific aim. It marks the transition from being stable in the vertical plane to becoming fluid in the sagittal plane (moving back and forth). The rhythm originates in the urethral sphincter muscle initiating the flow of urine. Typical activities in this phase include chasing and catching games.

Urethral Run–Stop–Go. During the second half of the third year of life, children learn to initiate and stop the flow of urine as well as to stop themselves while running, without falling. Movement qualities develop an abrupt sharpness that has an urgent or impatient sense of time. Favorite activities include squirting water and stop–start games such as musical chairs and red–light–green–light.

Inner-Genital Phase. The inner-genital phase is the developmental stage beginning in the fourth year of life and the task is to integrate past and present needs. Children become interested in the inner wavy sensations stemming from their internal pelvic organs. They are also interested in babies and playing with dolls in a nurturing fashion. Typically they alternate between mature behavior and regression to earlier, more disorganized patterns. Both girls and boys begin nagging and are unclear about what they require to satisfy their needs.

Outer-Genital Phase

The outer-genital phase is the developmental stage between the fifth and seventh years of life. The task is to become outwardly directed, with increased needs for gross motor activity and intensified relationships. Movements in this phase are intense, percussive, and abrupt, as in jumping and leaping, and originate in the outer genitals.

Even normal children in any phase of development may regress, at times, in order to sense the mastery that they achieved in the previous phase. Temporary regression is often a sign of resilience when children become overwhelmed by current developmental challenges. The case material below traces relevant portions of the developmental sequence outlined previously. An overview of KMP clinical concepts is in order before the case itself, however.

Dance/movement therapists have been involved in the treatment of autistic children for decades (Adler, 1968; Blau & Siegel, 1978; Kalish, 1968; Levy, 1988). For an extensive discussion of autism see Erfer, Chapter 14.

The Case of Warren

Background

Warren was a 4-year-old, fragile-looking boy with a fair complexion, who was neatly dressed, cautious, and timid. He had been diagnosed as autistic. Warren's characteristic behaviors included: withdrawal, passivity, minimal eye contact, toe walking, ritualistic perseverations, rocking, head banging, and no verbal language. Tests indicated no neurological impairment. Warren was attending a private, special educational day school where I saw him twice a week for ½ hour sessions over a 7 month period. The sessions were held in a large carpeted room containing gross motor equipment, mats, and a small box of wooden instruments. Soft music was often played. The room was arranged in the same way for each session to maintain a consistent and predictable environment. In addition, two other therapists worked individually with autistic boys in the same room at the same time as Warren's sessions. This arrangement allowed for the possibility of peer interaction.

Establishing a Relationship

First Session: The goals were to support Warren's exploration of the new environment, to initiate a relationship, to observe his movement patterns, and to move with him. To this latter end, I did not always move exactly as Warren moved, instead I tried to **"attune"** to or match his patterns of muscular tension and release in order to create a feeling of empathy. Early in the session Warren began to spin and bounce a balloon, showing little interest in me. When I mirrored his movements with another balloon, he seemed oblivious. When he began to march around the space, I marched beside him, noticing that he maintained no eye contact. In an effort to make eye contact, I faced Warren and created a vertical wall with my body, not allowing him to pass. At that moment of confrontation, Warren looked directly at me.

At this point, Michael, one of the other children in the session, walked between us. Immediately Warren lay down and exposed his teeth, perhaps angry that Michael had intruded. The two boys began to wrestle, and Warren pushed and kicked with **high intensity** and **vehemence**[1]. The other therapist and I separated the children and held them firmly while saying, "We won't let you hurt each other." The goal at this point was to redirect the aggressive energy into creative outlets, which used similar energy patterns; I reintroduced the balloon. An interaction of sounds that were intense in nature, matching the intensity of Warren's earlier aggressive movements, gradually developed.

Developing Assertive Movement Qualities

Second Session: When Warren arrived late to the session, Michael and Kenny, the other boys, were already involved. Warren first stamped on the mat angrily with **vehemence** and **high intensity**, and I duplicated these qualities in both muscle tension and body shape. Michael seemed pleased to see Warren and immediately went over to him. In response, Warren opened his mouth to bare his teeth. He resisted Michael's advances by standing still and maintaining a constant, rigid level of muscle tension,[2] an immature form of aggression that had no effect on Michael. The stamping movements Warren used in the previous session reflected a more mature form of aggression. It appeared that in a relationship, Warren was not able to express himself effectively. I patted the two boys on the back and said, "Michael wanted to say hello to Warren, but Warren wasn't ready yet."

Third Session: When Warren arrived, he started marching around the mat. I marched next to him, but he did not respond. In order to create more possibility for eye contact, I began to walk in front of Warren and to follow his movements while facing him. Warren smiled when he saw his motions mirrored back. When Michael entered the room, the two boys lay down together on the mat. This time Warren smiled instead of showing his teeth. For a brief moment, they seemed to recognize each other.

Warren left the mat to climb on the bars and began to shake them vigorously. Climbing is a motor skill that develops in the **anal phase**. I faced Warren and developed a "shaking the bars" game in which we both rocked toward and away from each other in the same rhythm. Warren maintained eye contact during the game and smiled, which seemed to indicate that the **attunement** helped facilitate interaction. He later put his finger on my smiling cheek and pushed it down using an **anal straining rhythm**.[3] Our relationship was beginning to develop; a feeling of connection and mutuality was established. When he reached for a ring on the bars that he couldn't quite get, I put out my hand and Warren took it. When he indicated that he wanted to come down, I carried him off the bar.

He lay flat in my arms, but he did not allow his muscles to relax. His body tension reflected that he was cautious about allowing me to support him.

Anal Phase Development

Sessions 4 through 14: During these sessions Warren continued to develop his relationships with me and with Michael. The movement patterns exhibited continued to progress within the **anal phase**.

In one session the two boys were able to be in the playhouse together without fighting. In another session, they took turns going up the ladder. Warren also began to assert himself. He used **strength** to keep Michael away. For example, when Michael tried to take a tire that Warren was using, Warren pushed Michael.

With regard to the development of our relationship, there were the inklings of playfulness, developing trust, and testing limits. Warren began to make new faces and sounds and initiated a teasing game of "take-away" with a toy telephone and another game of "peek-a-boo." He became more adventurous in his climbing and practiced sliding on and off a barrel into my arms. Once Warren tried to open the closet door. When told not to, he made deep sounds and appeared frustrated. His response was to sit on the mat using rigid movements (**bound even flow**). I sat next to him and said, "You are angry because I won't let you go into the closet." The next time I prevented him from opening the closet, he stomped over to the ladder and shook it **vehemently**. The stomping and shaking expressed his anger outwardly, a progressive step along the developmental line. I reinforced Warren's anger by stating it in words.

During these sessions, Warren began to use movement qualities in the **vertical plane**, the plane most often used in the **anal phase**. For example, at times he picked himself up and plopped down on the mat or climbed up and down the bars and reached out for assistance. Once when Warren became interested in some small bean bags, he threw them down hard on the ground in an **anal straining rhythm**.

Movement Patterns of Self-Defense

Fifteenth Session: There was a breakthrough that showed itself in Warren's ability to use appropriate self-defense patterns. Warren was playing with a blue piece of paper and the climbing bars. He meticulously put the paper around one bar. When Michael took the paper, Warren walked away in an avoidance pattern, **channeling** his attention to the door and ignoring Michael. To encourage Warren, I picked him up, brought him over to Michael and helped him retrieve the paper. He then collapsed on the mat and began to cry. I told him it was all right for him to get the paper and stroked his arm. The words and reassuring touch seemed to calm him and he stopped crying. He looked at me, began to circle around the mat and stopped to see if I was moving with him. Satisfied with my nonverbal response, he smiled. The next time Michael touched the blue paper, Warren held onto it, using **high intensity, even flow and strength,**[4] indicating that he was now able to hold on to his possession, using healthy aggressive movements.

Sixteenth Session: I gave Warren more space today and used **attunement** to match his tension qualities. Positioned further away from him than usual, I provided support but allowed more autonomy. There continued to be more eye contact and Warren began using new quick, short, high sounds while marching around the mat.

Seventeenth Session: Warren displayed several instances of assertive and related behavior. He was able to stand up to Michael who tried to intrude while Warren was exploring a rollosphere (a large, round piece of equipment designed for children to get into and roll around in). Later in the session, when Warren stamped on the mat, I duplicated his sounds by patting the mat. He watched me most of the time, smiled and initiated a new pattern of rolling away from and toward me. It appeared that by not imitating his movements exactly (not stamping next to him but reflecting in sound), he was able to experiment with new interactions.

Eighteenth Session: Warren and I continued with this newly developing ritual in which I patted the mat in rhythm to his changing gaits. He then became interested in four sticks, which he put up in a row and then proceeded to knock down, continuing the **anal straining phase** theme of up–down verticality. He again stood up for himself by holding on to the sticks when Michael tried to take them.

Nineteenth Session: Warren experimented with new ways of using the sticks, tapping my sticks with his, and varying the intensity of contact, using **light**[5] and forceful qualities. He also allowed me to support his back while he climbed higher on the bars, and reached out for help to climb down. In this session, Warren was able to use adaptive movement patterns, accept support, and again he asserted himself.

Twentieth Session: When Warren came in, he went directly to the box of instruments containing the wooden sticks and sat down without looking at me. I sat to the side of him and, as he played the instruments briefly, I tried to parallel his sounds. He became interested in the box itself, flicking the top flap with his thumb, a behavior that he had exhibited in the past with pieces of paper. I flicked with him, but Warren appeared indifferent. He glanced at me briefly.

I began to rub his back to the rhythm he used while flicking the box and for the first time, Warren lay down on my lap and released his weight. He responded well to this specific form of **tension-flow attunement** called **touch attunement.**[6]

Creating A Movement Ritual

Twenty-first Session: This session was a turning point in our relationship. Warren began marching around the mat, his shoulders tense and raised, his body rigid in **bound flow.** He lifted his knees and thumped his feet and vocalized a short "e" sound every time he stepped down. I duplicated his marching rhythm and joined him in the "e" sounds. He noticed the sounds, smiled, and changed his march to quick, short runs. I matched the changes. While changing from running to marching to running again, Warren watched to make sure I was following. He looked, turned away, squinted, and laughed playfully. I did the same.

Warren then changed the pattern of circling to running away from the circle and returning to a spot near my back. He turned around, squinted, laughed, and ran back to me. As he left the circle, I began to lean back to look at him, at which point he laughed again. I lay back every time Warren left the circle and came back to sitting when he returned. This developed into a circle ritual.

Through this action, I responded to Warren's change in pattern with a similar change. I decided to remain lying down in order to see how Warren would react. He approached and when I didn't get up, he put his hand on my knee in a gesture that seemed to indicate that he wanted me to sit. When I did so Warren laughed and made eye contact. Our pattern developed. Warren ran to the corner, I lay down, then he ran back and touched my knee to get me to sit up. When it was time for the session to end, I offered Warren my hand. We marched hand in hand back to the classroom making "e" sounds and smiling.

This was the first time Warren showed some continued awareness of me through consistent eye contact, smiling, and touch. A new trust seemed to develop that allowed Warren to take initiative and exert some control over the environment. When I duplicated his rhythm instead of his movement Warren responded more creatively.

Twenty-second Session: After first returning to the circle ritual Warren then went over to the bars. As he climbed, I supported his back, and he reached for me to carry him down. He continued to climb when the other children came by and did not leave as he had done before. For the first time, he climbed with the other children and trusted himself to be caught as he fell into my arms. He then began to walk around the room, to explore the window, the light, and the door. He was beginning to progress to the next phase of development, the **urethral running phase.**

Twenty-fourth Session: The session began with the circle ritual, which included a fair amount of touch. At the bars, Warren reached out for me to spin him around, and he continued to make eye contact and smile. With help from me he tried to hang on the bars.

Transition to the Urethral Phase

Twenty-fifth Session: The session again began with the circle ritual. There was an added change when Warren stepped quickly near my head several times, using a **urethral run–stop–go rhythm**.[7] He was beginning to add qualities of the next phase of development, the **urethral phase**, seen in normal child development between the ages of 2 and 3. It is important to note that as the child begins to integrate movement qualities of the phase he is in, qualities from the next phase appear in his movement repertoire.

Warren also went up the bars completely on his own in this session. This is an indication that he had mastered the ability to climb, which is crucial for the **anal straining phase**. In keeping with his transition to the next phase, Warren ran and changed his speed from slow to fast. This reflected his interest in timing. At one point he walked in slow motion, a totally new time quality for Warren. He ran back and forth over to the windows, tapped, and then ran over to the bars where he leaned back in my arms and indicated he wanted to be spun around. His new interest in timing and sagittal motion (i.e., moving forward and backward) were indications that he was making a wholehearted transition to the next phase.

While he was on the bars his shoe came off, and he played a game in which he did not allow me to tie his shoe but pulled away his foot and laughed in a teasing way. During this session, he appeared more spontaneous. His movement qualities included the indulgent efforts, **indirectness**,[8] **lightness**, and **deceleration**.[9] He seemed to show more trust in me and in his own ability. We marched back to his classroom singing.

Twenty-sixth Session: Warren initiated more variety and less adherence to set structures. His vocalizations seemed like gibberish instead of the usual single syllable repetition and included more variation in sounds. He climbed on the bars and jumped off for the first time, imitating Kenny. He was much more aware of the other children in the room. In keeping with the free flowing **urethral running phase**, he ran around the room in a less defined way, embracing this new quality. He played running and chasing games with me and the children in the room. I supported Warren's new movements by running with him and by helping him structure the games.

Another fluid pattern occurred when he began to experiment with moving his hands and arms in floating motions. Together, we synchronized in the flowing dance of the **urethral phase**.

Spontaneity

Twenty-seventh Session: During this session, there was more spontaneous interaction. We began by briefly engaging in the circle ritual. At the bars, Warren jumped off with Kenny and smiled a good part of the session. He initiated a game in which we put our hands together and then pulled them apart, perhaps in response to the termination[10] process that had recently begun. He sought more physical contact, signaling that he wanted me to spin him around and carry him.

Twenty-eighth Session: There was a continuation of spontaneous interaction between us. Warren appeared to understand verbal cues and he was able to relax when held, carried, and spun. The session began with a short version of the circle ritual, quickly followed by a climb on the bars. He stood up on the top bar, a new challenge, and jumped into my arms, more willing to take a risk. He began spontaneous hand gestures, which developed as he maintained eye contact. He put his hands on his cheeks, knees and neck, while I named the body parts. At the end of the session, we moved playfully around each other on the mat. This broke the rigid circling patterns and was an indication of his new ability to form a mutual and spontaneous relationship.

Discussion

The processes of **attunement** and **adjustment** enhance every therapist's ability to make clinical choices. **Attunement** is based on a sharing of qualities of muscle tension, and **shape-flow adjustment** is based on a similarity of breathing patterns and shape of the body between individuals. They represent nonverbal expressions of empathy and trust, respectively (Kestenberg, 1985b). A consistent "holding environment" (Winnicott, 1965) and a sense of continuity were created in the therapy by sameness over time both in the physical layout of the room and in the consistent presence of other therapists and children.

One of the more dramatic aspects of this case was the development of movement rituals, which established a predictable form within which a relationship could be structured. In the KMP model, predictability provides the form in which trust can flourish. Creativity, spontaneity, and emotional dynamics can all be contained within a consistent structure. Warren was able to relate within the safety of the ritual, until he was ready to try new and spontaneous patterns. These rituals were created initially when I matched rhythmic sounds to the beat of his marching movements. The rituals became more elaborate as the sessions progressed and then began to diminish as he was able to establish the beginning stages of a genuine interaction.

The KMP approach furthered an understanding of the sequence of movement phases typical in development and enabled me to provide a suitable environment in which the developmental process could evolve. I altered my approach to Warren in accordance with his needs. Although Warren was 4, he was functioning primarily in the **anal straining phase** of development, typical of an 18-month-old child. In the course of treatment, he began to make a transition to the next phase of development—the **urethral phase**. He became more fluid and mobile in his movements.

As the course of treatment progressed, Warren showed fewer autistic symptoms and related more spontaneously. The maturation of his movement patterns enabled him to have a greater impact on his environment. Initially his expression of anger was limited to showing his teeth, which had little or no effect on the other children. As the therapy continued, he used more adaptive movements and showed his feelings more overtly. Toward the end of treatment he demonstrated an improved ability to handle his aggression and his relationships with the other boys.

16

The "4's": A Dance Therapy Program for Learning-Disabled Adolescents

Diane Duggan

This chapter describes a dance therapy program for learning-disabled adolescents and the development of a movement structure that engaged the youth and met their needs both as adolescents and as persons with learning disabilities. Two case studies will illustrate gains made by participants over the course of time.

It is important for all dance therapists to consider the use of structure in our work. Structure is always present, whether it is obvious, as in groups for severely retarded children, or more subtle, as in the framework of the witness in authentic movement (Levy, 1988). In order to use structure most fruitfully, we must acknowledge its presence and relate its form and degree to the needs of our clients.

Structure helps to create a "holding environment," a time and space in which clients can feel safe enough to be themselves. The term "holding environment" derives from Winnicott's (1965) description of the conditions necessary for emotional development. In the normal course of development the mother or other caretaker provides these conditions for the infant. In the therapeutic setting they are provided by the clinician.

A dance therapy session structure serves several functions vital to the therapeutic process. As stated above, structure "holds" the client, providing an environment in which he or she is safe and free to respond. This promotes the trust that is the sine qua non of a therapeutic relationship. Structure also "holds" the movement. Because movement is transitory it is easily lost; structure enables movement phrases, images, and insights to coalesce, preventing their energy and meaning from dissipating. This allows for the acknowledgment of the client's experience as well as for the possibility of further exploration and development of what has transpired.

Structure in a dance therapy session can be provided through rhythm, spatial formation, interaction patterns, music, rituals, props, images, or signals. The amount and kind of structure will vary with the developmental level of clients and should be consonant with their needs and interests.

Structure is a dynamic, interactive concept, not a static one. It develops within the interaction between the therapist and the client and should be flexible enough to accommodate a range of possibilities in this relationship. Although I will discuss a specific, concrete structure below, it is important not to apply it as a formula for all adolescents. The structure a dance therapist employs must evolve from the interaction of his/her experience and training with an understanding of the needs of the clients both on a theoretical level and as expressed in their verbal and nonverbal communications.

Development of the Structure

I began the dance therapy program described here in September 1979 at a public high school for learning-disabled adolescents. The school was comprised of approximately 250 special education students, the majority of whom were male. The students ranged in age from 14 to 21 and came primarily from economically disadvantaged backgrounds. Most were African American with a large Hispanic minority. Although of normal intelligence, the students had severe learning problems and lacked basic reading and math skills. Many were dyslexic, and most had attention deficits. All of the students had severe problems with self-esteem, likely due in large part to feelings of incompetence and histories of repeated failure in school. Most exhibited inadequate social skills and behavior problems, and they had difficulties interacting with their peers.

Traditionally, dance therapy with learning-disabled children has concentrated on movement activities designed to develop body image, balance, spatial awareness, coordination, memory, impulse control, and socialization (Duggan, 1981). However, the usual game-like format used to address these areas can be experienced by adolescents as infantilizing. With this in mind, I began with a Chaceian circle to structure the group, intending to concentrate on socialization and emotional expression and to work indirectly on the other areas. To my dismay, the circle continuously flattened out into a line. At first I patiently regrouped into a circle, only to have the participants fall firmly back into lines. The meaning of this behavior was initially unclear, but it was obviously important.

Part of the problem seemed to center around adolescent ambivalence toward self display. On the one hand teenagers are exhibitionistic, wanting to be attended to and admired; on the other hand, because of uncertainty about their developing identity, they crave anonymity and deindividuation in a group. A circle exposes everyone to everyone else; there is no place to hide. The lines the teenagers insisted on forming seemed a safer formation for them. In their line, group members were not directly confronted by each other, yet they were supported on either side by peers, with whom they could relate in parallel to whatever transpired.

The peer group is vital to adolescents (Erikson, 1968), and by definition it does not include adults as equal members. A circle is inclusive and nonhierarchical; all members are, at least potentially, on equal footing. The lines the teens persisted in forming seemed to symbolize not only the solidarity of their peer group but, also, their differentiation from and opposition to me, the authority figure. Their everyday experience in the classroom afforded them the security of a linear, hierarchical arrangement. However, in the initial dance therapy sessions I was asking them to risk something new involving body movement and self-disclosure in full view of their peers and in full collaboration with me.

After several days of circles flattening into lines, I honored the teens' nonverbal request and told them to line up. They did so with enthusiasm. There was an immediate transformation, and, although some resistance remained, they became decidedly more relaxed. I had accepted the position of authority and "otherness," which they needed me to hold. It is a paradox that from this act, which initially seemed distancing and uncomfortable, there arose an intimacy based on the familiarity and predictability of our respective roles. The adolescents needed me to be clearly differentiated from them; only in that way could they start to trust me to "hold" them, to organize and set limits so that they could begin to feel safe.

Although I had accepted and confirmed the new order, questions persisted about what the group was supposed to be doing. I had originally told them that they were dancing together to get in touch with their feelings and to examine and work through issues that arose among them. Needless to say, that was not a satisfactory answer, and questions persisted. They needed a concrete goal; just being in the here and now was much too threatening. When someone suggested that they put on a show at Christmas, the group instantly seized on the idea. They needed a format that gave limits and a feeling of purpose; the idea of working toward a show met some of those needs.

The immediate question (after what they would wear) was what they would do. Although I tried to enlist their ideas, offering various frameworks for improvisation, they were unsure and not ready to commit. Acutely aware of their demand for me to provide for them, I responded by choosing a Ghanaian "highlife," a swingy musical style popular in West African social dancing, which they liked. I carefully worked out combinations at home every night to "feed" to them the next day. Invariably these combinations were rejected. They were "too hard," "too easy," too much mine and not enough theirs. We reworked the ideas together and struggled slowly through the choreography. Although it provided a focus for the group, it was somewhat limited and artificial.

I felt caught in a dilemma. The group obviously needed structure, but the simple format I was providing seemed inadequate, and the group members were as yet too mistrustful to contribute overtly to the process. The group needed a structure, not to restrict them but to set them free. An ideal structure would engage and organize them and address prominent adolescent issues, such as identification with the peer group and sexuality. It would be definite enough to support them but also flexible and responsive to their needs.

I soon hit on an idea that was so simple that it didn't even present itself as an idea at the time. While trying to come up with the next step in the choreography I found myself dancing in a "holding pattern" of four beats to the right (step, step, step, tap) and four to the left (step, step, step, tap). This kept the movement flowing and the group moving together. This pattern derived from my study of Haitian dance with Jean-Léon Destiné, who introduced Haitian dance as an art form in the United States (Terry, 1956).

The pattern proved compelling to the group. When they asked what it was called, I simply responded "4's." Thus the "4's" were born. This proved to be the perfect holding environment, engaging and simple enough to be within the grasp of all of them, yet challenging in that it initially required attention to learn.

It is worthwhile noting that this structure arose spontaneously, almost unconsciously, in a moment of nonverbal rapport in the ongoing dialogue between my unconscious and that of the group members. I had been trying to organize myself, but the group members recognized in my actions the organization that they also needed.

Although captivated by the step, some group members initially had trouble with the final "tap" in the four-beat sequence. Because of their impulsivity they tended to commit their weight in a step on the last beat. This obviated any further choice, forcing them to continue in the same direction. The 4's structure was based on "free flow" (Laban, 1960), loose, unrestricted muscle action, which was bracketed on the fourth beat by "bound" (Laban, 1960) pauses in which movement was restricted. These bound pauses allowed the dancers to change direction, so that they could dance continuously in lines without over-running spatial boundaries and perseverating in a single direction.

In order to execute the step properly the group members had to bind their flow by tightening opposing muscle groups and controlling their movement, suspending the impulse to commit their weight on the final beat. The inability to do this was in fact, an embodiment of one of the most pervasive problems in the group, that of poor impulse control. The 4's step required them, not to deny the impulse to move, but to channel it into a gestural "lightness" (Laban, 1960) that did not commit their body weight: a tap as opposed to a step. The tap enabled them to preserve their options, becoming more flexible in directing their movements through space. It took some reflection and effort for these youngsters to achieve this. The challenge was real, but limited enough to over-come. Their mastery of it was a geniune accomplishment.

This small initial challenge was like an initiation rite, and once it was over-come all participants attained the privileged yet accessible status as a member of a cohesive group. The most compelling and meaningful aspect of the 4's was that it enabled them to move in unison, submerging individual fears and doubts in the certainty of group action. It was the perfect manifestation of the peer group: accessible but exclusive, "hip" but conforming.

The 4's structure was able to contain and organize many individual and group expressions of sexuality and aggression, such as the grinding of hips, stomping, and thrusting of arms. It withstood them all by subsuming even the most suggestive movements into its invariant convention of measured, precise symmetry. Within the structure of the 4's they were able to relax and be them-selves in the company of others. The 4's protected and supported them so that little by little they were able to simply be. No one asked about meaning any-more. The meaning was inherent in the structure: a unified group of competent adolescents who belonged, no longer isolated and no longer vulnerable.

The Use of Conventional Dance Steps

The 4's provided a rhythmic and spatial structure, but it was open as to con-tent and shape. There were three groups in total and each group developed vocabularies of 4's steps unique to their own needs. The adolescents offered many popular dance steps in this process. Among dance therapists there is con-troversy regarding the use of conventional dance steps, with some maintaining that these movements are inauthentic and keep individuals away from their feelings. I believe that to say that these movements are not authentic is to miss the point. As always in dance therapy, it is important to begin with what clients offer, rather than requiring them to attempt something unfamiliar.

Adolescent dance steps are both the expression of their sexual and agggressive urges and the defense against the acting out of these impulses (Group for the Advancement of Psychiatry, 1968). It is the stereotypic character of the movements that permits them to function as defenses, dictating shape, dynamics, and proxemics. These conventions clearly signal the dancer's intention to communicate and provoke rather than to consummate. The content of these movements also functions as an expression and communication of identity, both of subculture and gender. These steps were accepted as worthwhile contributions, valid expressions of self.

This use of adolescent dance steps is in some ways analogous to mirroring the stereotyped gestures of an autistic child. It establishes a bridge to the clients while permitting them the security and gratification of familiar movement patterns during the early, diffficult stages of establishing a relationship (Duggan, 1978).

These movements were transformed by the 4's structure into a means of self-expression and relating to others. This was a crucial process, for the group was well into its second year before the members became capable of more free-form, individualistic improvisation. The paradox that structure and stereotyped movement can permit freedom and authenticity mirrors the paradox that formalized roles can facilitate real relationships, as I had earlier discovered. The external order permits the expression of emotionally charged impulses because it contains the impulses and permits their control. Interaction is facilitated because attention is initially focused on form and roles rather than on personalities, thereby reducing self-consciousness and anxiety. The structure is both an organizing factor and a template for interaction, ordering experience and affording a safe opportunity for self-expression and satisfying contact.

In each of the groups the content of the 4's was slightly different, as was the music they brought to the sessions. I became the repository for these differences, reflecting back each group's uniqueness. In this way several distinctly different dances evolved, all based on the 4's. One group, comprised mainly of girls, developed variations based on sustained horizontal pelvic swings, giving their movements a swaying, sexy quality. Another, more aggressive group built a 4's vocabulary with quick, sagittal pelvic thrusts and strong, quick high-five hand slaps. The third group focused more on spatial patterns, building highly intricate sequences of direction changes. There was some competition among the groups, a reflection of the adolescents' concerns over issues of inclusion and exclusion. As the vocabulary of steps increased and became more sophisticated the teens began to feel the assurance and relative ease that only true competence can bring. They developed their coordination, spatial orientation, and balance as they mastered the group's repertoire of 4's variations.

Use of Performance

In the first weeks of the program, in response to the demands of group members for concrete goals, I had agreed to put on a show. Dance therapists are primarily interested in the process of their work, not its product, and it is unusual for them to produce shows. However, Marian Chace, one of the founders of dance therapy, frequently used performance in her work at St. Elizabeth's Hospital (Chaiklin, 1975). The idea of performance was compatible with the adolescent penchant for self-display, and it provided an acceptable forum for them to command attention and demonstrate their competence.

The precision of a group moving in synchrony is inherently pleasing to the beholder, and I knew that the success of the proposed show depended on ensuring that group members could dance in unison. Early in the development of the program I had begun to cultivate leadership of the 4's among group members. While I danced with them and "held" the sessions, providing the safe, facilitative environment, each of the teens had a chance to "hold" the dance together. The designated leader had to decide what to do next and tell the group members in a clear and timely fashion so that everyone had sufficient time to prepare to execute the steps. When done well, "calling" the dance produced fluent transitions and unison movement. It was very impressive to spectators, who were usually not aware of the leader's role in organizing the steps and communicating to the other dancers.

Each group had named the 4's steps they had invented, so that the leader could name a step and the group members would know what to do. The physical features of the room, its door, windows, fixed seats, and backstage wall were used as spatial referents. The leader could give a direction to "chase" at the door and everyone knew that one line would move toward the other while the other line retreated, and that this movement would begin at the side of the stage closest to the door.

When the leader was not able to communicate his or her instructions to other members, the group literally fell apart. As various group members tried on the role of leader, the followers were encouraged to verbalize their feelings about the care the leader gave. In this process they learned how to say when they were not being adequately cared for by the leader, and some of the group members learned how to take care of the group.

Once the issue of my separateness had been resolved I had resumed dancing with the group, in their lines. Although it would not have been appropriate for me to dance in the show, they needed help to stay together. I began to sit at the foot of the stage in sessions, saying "...5, 6, 7, 8" to ensure everyone got off on the right beat. As a safety net there was a reliable holding pattern, the basic 4's walk, to return to whenever there was uncertainty. Its simple, wave-like periodicity quickly organized even the most chaotic mistakes.

In addition to the 4's, the steady, rhythmic beat of the music was a powerful organizing factor. We used music brought in by group members because it engaged them and gave them a sense of ownership in the sessions. Rap music was just becoming popular, and its hypnotic pulse fueled the dances. Misogynistic and otherwise objectionable lyrics gave rise to discussions about how males and females relate to each other. Again and again, the problems of mistrust and mutual exploitation arose.

In the last weeks before the show the structure of performance became a crucible. Important issues boiled to the surface and sought resolution. Primary was the anticipation of failure, which evoked the terror of public humiliation. All of the members had experienced failure in the past; that was why they had been placed in this school.

Issues of gender and of inclusion/exclusion became the battleground for the more primitive fears of the group. The girls closed ranks and began to berate the boys. The boys, in turn, were only too ready to drop out as a way of dealing with their anxiety. Fortunately, there is always much to do in a stage production, and various "crew" jobs, such as lighting, D.J., and gaffer went to the boys. I recognized that the division of labor along stereotypical gender lines was reassuring to the group members. It allowed them to devote their energies to their respective tasks rather than becoming distracted by sexual tensions on the stage.

The adolescents were not the only ones anxious at the prospect of the coming show. I was worried and disheartened by their acting out. A few weeks before the performance I dreamed I was slogging across a wide river carrying a large, Santa Claus-like sack on my back. It was extremely heavy, and the going was slow and arduous. In the bag were the group members, screaming like babies, frightened of the journey, but needing to cross to the other side. I felt strongly that if I could only keep the heavy, writhing load together and deliver them to the other side, the next time some of them would be walking beside me, helping to carry others. The key was the sack, the structure that held them together and would enable me to transport them to their own authentic success.

Other members of the school community rallied to the effort: The metal shop built stage lights, the graphics shop designed and silkscreened a "Foxy

Mommas" logo for one group's costume sweatshirts, the photography shop took pictures of the groups and prepared to shoot the performance, and the sewing teacher assisted dancers in sewing skirts for the highlife number. Because of body-image issues and lack of funds the costumes for two of the dances consisted of sweatshirts and jeans.

The show was a great success. We presented three dances, using lighting and simple costumes to transcend the limits of the small, bare platform stage. The most impressive factor, for the dancers and the audience alike, was the fact that the groups danced in unison, thanks to the supportive, flexible structure of the 4's. Students in the photography class documented the dancers' triumph, and I displayed the photos on the bulletin boards. Students from throughout the school came to pore over the photos, but none so regularly as the dancers themselves. As time went on, this was especially true after an absence or some crisis in their lives. Doubting themselves they sought confirmation of their achievement in the photos.

In subsequent years of the dance therapy program, the 4's remained dominant as the basic organizing structure in sessions. It reached its choreographic apotheosis in an elaborate, sophisticated number in the second Christmas show. This dance was based on a syncopated 4's variation that celebrated the dancers' mastery of the genre. The hesitation step marked a resurgence of the impulse control issue and a demonstration of the dancers' mastery of it. After that the 4's figured only skeletally in choreography for shows but was still vital in sessions, where I continued to use it as a way of integrating new people and enabling the entire group to dance together.

In the third year we performed at a children's psychiatric hospital. We presented a program called "The Beat," which used a rap narrative about rhythm and dance and integrated African, modern, jazz, and breakdance. In the finale the rap stressed that the beat of life is in us all, and the dancers performed a 4's-based dance. They then called up children from the audience and taught them the basic 4's step, incorporating them into the performance. The group had come a long way, from being dependent on the structure of the 4's to using it to hold and nurture others; the 4's had been equal to the challenge.

Male–Female Duets

The success of the first Christmas show had demonstrated the reliability of the 4's structure and provided a sense of independence and self mastery that permitted the group to begin dealing more directly with two major themes, sexuality and aggression. After the Christmas vacation the males reasserted their equality as dancers, causing two important innovations, which addressed precisely those themes. The first was a male–female duet. Most of the Hispanic male group members liked to hustle, but they seldom had female partners. For one thing, the ratio of males to females in the school was 10 to 1, and most of the girls either did not care to hustle or did not know how. I did not make myself available as a hustle partner because it was too sexualizing, and confusion as to the nature of my availability might lead to anxiety and mistrust. The Hispanic boys solved the problem of the lack of female partners by dancing with each other. In spite of their strong tradition of machismo, or maybe because of it, they partnered each other with considerable grace and without apparent self-consciousness.

One of the boys, Ferdie, wanted to perform a hustle in the spring show. He asked Lisa, an African-American girl who did not know how to hustle but was willing to learn, and he taught her. This was significant both for his maturity in reaching out to her and for the bold step across ethnic lines that it represented. There was often tension between the two ethnic groups; Ferdie and Lisa's dance, to a song called "Romeo and Juliet," made a statement of acceptance and raised the possibility of intergroup romance. It was purely an artistic partnership, as they were not boyfriend and girlfriend. I contributed to their effort by teaching them partnering techniques and various dramatic poses to theatricalize the dance. The group talked a lot about support and holding as we worked on the dance. At this point it was hard for anyone in the group to take this concept past gender stereotypes, but it marked a vast improvement over their original exploitative and potentially hostile stance.

Ferdie and Lisa's dance was based on the hustle, a socially acceptable way for teens to dance at the time. It began a tradition of partnering that was further developed the following autumn in a modern *pas de deux* set to a contemporary ballad. This was a significant step forward, as it marked the teens' willingness to transcend conventional adolescent dance forms. After its success, many of the boys were willing to work on and perform dances with female partners in various styles, ranging from modern to balletic to jazz. In the third year of the program so many boys wanted to participate in a *pas de deux* that I choreographed a group dance for three couples. It became increasingly acceptable for boys and girls to dance in a supportive, considerate manner. Several *danseurs nobles* emerged, boys who partnered with grace and integrity. Dances passed into the program's repertoire and were taught to newcomers by experienced group members.

It is interesting to note that the boys and girls danced as partners almost exclusively in the choreography and performance portions of the sessions. They did not partner in the freer-form dancing that made up much of the sessions, where the 4's still dominated. This relegation of partnering to choreography and performance gave it more structure, thus lessening the inevitable anxiety and sexual tension that develop when teenage girls and boys touch and move in synchrony at close range. The partner dances, while often sensitive, had a mildly detached quality, as the partners concentrated on their steps. This focus on the structure of the dance can be viewed as a mechanism that helped them tolerate the potentially stimulating interaction with a partner, while at the same time developing that interaction.

Breakdance

Another significant contribution in the first year of the program came from the African-American males. Just after the Christmas show a boy who was not in the program asked me if freestyle dancing could be included in the next show. Unsure about what he meant, I asked for a demonstration. He brought his friends, and they performed dynamic, athletic improvisations with each other, striving throughout to outdo each other. I began to include it in sessions, and a whole new group of boys signed up. One boy, a member of a group called the Zulu Nation, described how gangs met and rumbled in dance instead of fighting. This was truly art as sublimation! The first spring show included a breakdance exhibition, which was a dazzling psychodrama of stylized aggression and one-upmanship. The boys fought for ownership of the stage, but the formalization of their aggressive impulses transformed it from acting out into a work of art.

The breakdancers evolved over the years from a loosely organized aggregate of competitive and highly individualistic dancers to a cohesive unit. During the second year they began doing partner work, using each others' bodies as spring boards for gymnastic feats and supporting each other in comic "freezes." In the third year breakdance numbers began with a dramatic choreographed entrance that proclaimed competition but which was in fact highly interactive and cooperative. The break dancers also began to support each other by clapping time in unison as a background for solo displays.

Both the hustle duet and the breakdancing opened new avenues of interaction and expression for the group. The duet started a tradition of male–female dancing that included support and caring, rather than exploitation. The breakdance brought in the commitment and energy of a group of males who tended to be more aggressive and competitive and gave them an avenue for self-expression and demonstration of their masculinity.

In the spring of the first year of the program we went on to perform at the New York City Very Special Arts Festival. Under the rules, we could only present one dance, but it could be 20 minutes long. Not wanting to exclude any-one, I took bits and pieces of five dances from the Christmas and spring shows and connected them with a rhyme, modeled after the hip-hop rap music we used in sessions. It integrated the hustle duet, breakdancers, an Afro-Caribbean dance, and two 4's-based dances. On the basis of their performance, the group was cho-sen to attend the New York Statewide Very Special Arts Festival, staying overnight at the Statler Hotel and attending a special banquet. This accomplish-ment was a powerful confirmation of the adolescents' self worth, and it enabled them for the first time to talk frankly about their handicaps. The group discussed the fact that the festival was for people with disabilities, like themselves. When they compared themselves with the other festival participants, many of whom were severely disabled, they were able to appreciate their relative strengths and to see themselves as competent people, a new experience for them.

Case Illustrations

Going into the program's second year the group was strong and resilient enough to allow for the exploration of individual issues. Two interrelated case examples illustrate different ways in which the adolescents used the sessions to work through problems and meet their needs.

"Trudy"

Trudy was known around the school as manipulative and exploitative, trading sexual favors for drugs, presents, and cash. Many teachers disliked her, perhaps threatened by her aggressive use of sexuality. Trudy had lived in a series of fos-ter homes since infancy, and although she longed for closeness, her basic phi-losophy was to get all she could from others before they abandoned her.

Trudy was cautious and bound in her movements, defensively peripheral and unable to give of herself. She caught on quickly to dance sequences and remembered them, however, which made her a good leader. She enjoyed the structure of the 4's and her mastery of its variations. The dance therapy ses-sions afforded her a unique opportunity to be recognized for her abilities and to be a sanctioned leader rather than the opponent of the teacher. Although she was not yet able to express her needs, developing her leadership ability was useful in getting her to attend to the needs of others, and she took her respon-sibility seriously. In her first semester in the program she participated in group dances, but after Christmas I began to work with her on a dance that expressed her relationships with males. Trudy worked from the outside in, not using movement expressively, but relating to song lyrics and carefully but dispassionately executing movements we choreographed together. Her dance was a sexy jazz number in which she "controlled" two of the boys, commanding them to react to her with flicks of her wrist and pointing gestures. The dance was based on Trudy's natural movement repertoire, so that she used distal parts of her body and did not involve her torso. The peripheral nature of her movement suggested an emotional distancing and lack of commitment, and was a clear expression of her psychological noninvolvement in relationships. Throughout the dance the boys took turns literally supporting and uplifting her; they ended by carrying her regally off the stage on their shoulders. As we choreographed, I discussed Trudy's role in the dance with her, leading to an acknowledgement of her need for control and recognition and the possibility of achieving these without hurting herself or others.

We acquired some costumes from another dance therapist, among them a pink satin tank leotard. None of the other girls felt ready to wear it, but Trudy was intrigued. She went to the bathroom with the other girls to try it on. When they returned they were all murmuring that she looked like Miss America. She proclaimed with amazement that she did indeed look like Miss America. I agreed and suggested that we keep the costume a secret in order to make more of an impact at the show. Trudy seemed to enjoy this period of symbolic chastity almost as much as the moment when she appeared in the show, to the appreciative applause of the audience.

In the following Christmas show Trudy became the first student to dance a free-form modern solo. Once again it was the theme of the song to which she initially related, rather than the expressive character of the movement. She was in love, and the song she chose spoke directly about the emptiness of exploitative relationships and the wonder of new-found passion. In choreographing the dance with her I included several Graham-like contractions, uncharacteristically postural and committed for her. Trudy performed these tentatively but with earnestness, trying on the new way of being. Her style of restricting her movement to peripheral body parts, which suggested defensiveness, was slowly giving way to postural involvement, an indication that she was becoming more in touch with her feelings and more committed to her actions.

The effect of the program on Trudy's self-esteem is reflected in a statement she made on a group outing to see the Alvin Ailey American Dance Theater. She started to rush impulsively across the street then drew back and said to me, "I have to take care of myself. I have to perform next week." Unfortunately Trudy's story does not have a totally happy ending. She became pregnant the following year, ready to live out her fantasy of having a family of her own. She dropped out of school and, unmarried and on welfare, eventually had three children. Trudy regarded her experience in the dance therapy program as a high point in her life, and years after leaving school she contacted me to find out where she could take dance classes and to ask for photographs of herself dancing so she could show her children.

"Tommy"

Trudy's story is intertwined with that of Tommy. Unlike Trudy, Tommy was creative and innocent in his openness to self-expression in dance, conveying grace and feeling in the unlikely form of a lanky, high-top sneakered boy. He came to school in December of 1980 and made his presence felt immediately. He was impossible to ignore, continually chased and grabbed by students or teachers in the hallway for taunting or otherwise provoking them. Tommy gravitated toward the dance therapy room, and although he was not programmed for dance therapy, I allowed him to participate in the upcoming Christmas show as a member of the lighting crew. During a rehearsal Tommy begged to be allowed to dance, and the breakdancers agreed to let him jam with them afterward. He was extraordinary! He showed great quickness, agility, and grace as he deftly and rather lewdly countered the best moves the other dancers could throw at him. At this point in the evolution of breakdancing this art form was decidedly a competitive, not a cooperative venture. Tommy's audacity and originality won the admiration of the other dancers, and they voted unanimously to include him in their number.

On the day of the show Tommy, wearing a silver lamé shirt, made an unforgettable entrance as he catapulted up onto the stage in a cartwheel and proceeded to demolish the opposition, "dogging" them with bold counters to their suggestive put-downs. The photography students documented his dazzling performance, and for weeks after students asked about the identity of this silver-shirted superstar, some refusing to believe that it was the ever-annoying Tommy.

Tommy joined the dance therapy group for two sessions a day, a joint request from both himself and most of the faculty. He was truly a wild child, a mixture of naiveté and impulsivity, relating only sporadically with sudden, often aggressive movements. Although he was a gifted dancer he could sustain the 4's dance only briefly and could not tolerate other interactive dances. He could participate fully only in breakdancing, a form that permitted him to dance as an individual, making only brief contact with others.

This began to change when he became interested in the tough, streetsmart Trudy. Tommy, who was only 15 and very inexperienced with girls, wanted to learn her jazz dance in order to be near her. He tried to learn one sequence, but in spite of his facility at picking up movements, he erroneously interpreted his role in a dip as throwing her down rather than supporting her. This was in keeping with the antisocial, aggressive nature of most of his contacts with others. Because of my habit of spotting any remotely risky moves and Trudy's well-honed survival instincts, she landed on her feet. But Tommy was humiliated, and he sat disconsolately in the back of the auditorium for the next hour, only confiding his sorrow and despair to me just before his double period was over. The next day we worked together on the move, and by the following day he had learned the entire dance to perfection.

In casting the spring performance that year I wanted Tommy to be in Trudy's dance. His dancing was graceful and full of feeling, and he desperately wanted to dance with Trudy. My aim was not to put on the most aesthetic production possible, however, but to make it a therapeutic experience. To this end I had made it a practice for the group to discuss and determine who would dance in what numbers. It had never seemed to backfire until then.

Trudy, with the support of the others, said she did not want Tommy in the dance. Tommy was anguished and began screaming and jumping around. I calmed him and suggested the group talk about it, privately not believing that any better resolution would come out of it. There followed a frank, caring discussion in which Trudy confronted Tommy with his unreliability and the fact that he constantly bedeviled and provoked people in the school. Surprisingly, Tommy was relieved, saying he'd been afraid Trudy hadn't wanted him because she thought he was stupid. Paul, one of Trudy's partners, told Tommy that if he could act more responsibly he'd be willing to let him take his place in the annual Very Special Arts Festival, which was to be held in May. Tommy's behavior did improve, especially in the dance therapy sessions. Not only did he take Paul's place at the Very Special Arts Festival, but he collaborated with me on the choreography for a lyrical, caring dance for himself and Trudy, which they performed at the June school awards ceremony. Tommy insisted that the principal come to witness his achievement.

Tommy constantly provoked the environment to take notice of him. He sought witnesses everywhere, nonverbally demanding that people attend to him. The performance aspect of the program was crucial to him, as it provided him with an acceptable device for commanding the attention of literally the whole school. Tommy's well-developed motor skills derived from a style of reacting to the environment through motility. His movements when he first came to the program were quick and aggressive. He repeatedly sought contact but was only able to provoke (and maybe only able to accept) aggressive responses from others. The dance therapy sessions required him to focus his movement and modulate its dynamics to permit participation and interaction with group members. His investment in dance and later his attraction to Trudy made it possible for him to be a part of the group and gradually to tolerate demands placed on him by the movement structures and by other group members. His change on a movement level, which enabled him to adapt to dance structures more rigorous than breakdancing, presaged his subsequent behavioral change. The following year he became the partner of choice in duets and other interactive dances with girls. This was due to his grace and skill and his developing ability to control his impulses.

Summary

The adolescents accomplished a great deal in the dance therapy program, both as a group and individually. They went from competitive, exploitative peer relationships to cooperative, mutually supportive interactions. Issues such as control of self and others, aggression, and sexuality were embodied in movement, enabling the teens to safely explore the meaning of these issues in their lives and to try on new ways of dealing with them.

At every step in the development of the program, I took my cues from the teens themselves. Training in human development and behavior guided me in working through their personal and age-specific concerns. I used dance to give shape and permanence to their movement expressions, gradually and interactively creating with them dances that were personally meaningful and pleasing.

The deceptively simple pattern of the 4's provided the initial structure, which brought the adolescents together and helped them to solidify into a group strong enough to withstand conflict and deal with important issues. It succeeded because it engaged them and provided a secure, age-appropriate structure with which to begin the difficult, rewarding work of self-discovery and change. It was resilient enough to grow as the group matured, initiating and supporting the ongoing development of individual members. In the end it affected their lives positively, enhancing their sense of competence and self-esteem and developing their ability to relate meaningfully and cooperatively with others.

Notes

1. Nameless: A Case of Multiplicity

1. My deepest gratitude goes to my mentor, Sidney Levy, Ph.D, (not a relative), for sharing with me his wisdom and compassion, and for encouraging me to write about this most unusual and important case. I would also like to thank Rachel for giving me the right to share our work. Finally, I would like to thank my three talented colleagues, Dr. Amy Schaffer, Dr. Nancy Schulman, and Jean Peterson, M.S.W., ATR, for their skill and sensitivity in their work with Rachel during the times that I had to be away from my practice.

2. This concept began with the pioneering work of M.A. Sechehaye (1951) and utilizes the patient's ability to experience symbolism as a kind of reality that can literally affect a change in the patient's thoughts and feelings. Sechehaye gave her patient an apple as a symbol for the breast to help the patient to stay connected to her, the therapist mother. A similar creative and symbolic use of the mind is illustrated in the case of Rachel.

3. Sidney Levy, Ph.D., Professor Emeritus New York University, originated LADS—the Levy Animal Drawing Story test in the 1940's. Levy is a Certified Psychologist and Psychoanalyst who is also a strong advocate for the arts in psychotherapy. LADS is taught along with other projective methods of assessment primarily in clinical psychology programs. It is the author's hope that these techniques will eventually be taught in creative-arts therapy programs and as part of the social work curriculum. Projectives are profoundly helpful as creative, diagnostic, and expressive tools. Under the tutelage of Dr. Sidney Levy, the author has been utilizing animal and figure drawing analysis as a part of ongoing assessment and creative movement expression in clinical practice with adults.

4. It is important to note that the use of self-disclosure is unusual in my practice. For Rachel, however, secrecy was profoundly threatening. For this reason, at her request, we spoke openly about the book and its contents.

3. Mobilizing Battered Women: A Creative Step Forward

1. Parts of the paper were previously published in the *American Journal of Dance Therapy 13*. (2) Fall/Winter 1991, under the title "Dance/Movement Therapy with Battered Women: A Paradigm of Action."

2. The clinical work described in this chapter is based on treatment in a shelter for women and therefore is written from that point of view. It is important to note, however, that the dynamics discussed are not limited to heterosexual or male-dominated relationships. Similar patterns of abuse may occur in any relationship.

3. The authors gratefully acknowledge the contributions of Karen Malpede for her creative collaboration in sessions with battered women. We also want to thank Eileen Moran, whose vision and support made this work possible.

5. Multiple Personality Disorder: A Group Movement Therapy Approach

1. Psychogenic fugues are sudden, unexpected, yet purposeful travel away from an accustomed locale with assumption of a new identity and an inability to recall one's past. Conversion symptoms are alterations or losses of physical functioning that suggest physical disorder, but are apparently expressions of psychological conflict or need (American Psychiatric Association, 1987).

7. Movement as Metaphor: Treating Chemical Addiction

1. The therapist should use this technique cautiously. It is usually not advisable to role-play a parent due to the intense negative emotions that this can prematurely trigger toward the therapist. When it is done, however, it is important to assess whether the patient can handle such a transference of feelings or whether it will be destructive to the therapeutic relationship.

8. Confronting Co-Dependency: Psychodramtic Movement Therapy Approach

1. Parts of this chapter were previously published in the *Arts in Psychotherapy* journal, 19, 1992, under the title of "Creativity and Change: The Two-Tiered Creative Art Therapy Approach to Co-dependency Treatment."

13. Early Intervention with Children at Risk for Attachment Disorders

1. Debi Karlinsky, C.S.W., DTR, provided some of the clinical material discussed in this chapter.

15. The Case of Warren: A KMP Approach to Autism

1. These two qualities are characteristic of the anal straining phase. High intensity is muscle tension that reaches extremely contracted or released levels, reflecting high excitation. Vehemence is a movement quality that attempts to impact the force of gravity through the use of high intensity of tension-flow, that is temper-tantrums.

2. He utilized *bound flow*, which is restrained muscle tension in which the agonist and antagonist muscles contract simultaneously, and *even flow*, which is muscle tension that is maintained at a constant level indicating rigidity or sameness. To produce *bound even flow*, the muscles are tensed internally and usually have no impact on the outside environment.

3. The *as* or *anal straining rhythm* is a movement pattern characterized by holding muscle tension at the same level for a prolonged length of time and then releasing it.

4. *Strength* is an adaptive movement pattern that serves as a fighting attitude toward gravity.

5. *Light* is a movement quality that serves as an indulgent or buoyant attitude toward gravity.

6. *Touch attunement* involves matching an individual's muscle tension through the process of touch. It can often be an effective way of making contact when other channels of communication fail.

7. The *urethral run–stop–go–rhythm* involves sharp movement qualities that start and end suddenly in the service of being able to stop and start running.

8. Indirectness is a movement quality that serves as an indulgent or multifocused attitude toward space.

9. Deceleration is a movement quality that serves as an indulgent or leisurely attitude toward time.

10. There would only be a few more sessions before the end of the school year.

Bibliography

Abt, L., & Bellak, L. (1950). *Projective psychology.* New York: Grove.

Adelson, E., & Fraiberg, S. (1974). Gross motor development in infants blind from birth. *Child Development, 45,* 114–126.

Adelson, E., & Fraiberg, S. (1976). Sensory deficit and motor development in infants blind from birth. In Z.S. Jastrzembska (Ed.) *The effects of blindness and other impairments on early development.* New York: American Foundation for the Blind.

Adler, G., & Buie, D.H. (1973). *The misuses of confrontation in the psychotherapy of borderline cases: Confrontation in psychotherapy.* In G. Adler & P.G. Myerson (Eds.). New York: Science House.

Adler, J. (1968). The study of an autistic child (film and presentation). *Proceedings of the American Dance Therapy Association, Third Annual Conference* (pp. 43–48). Madison, WI: American Dance Therapy Association.

Ainsworth, M. D. S., Blehar, M. C., Waters, E., & Hall, S. (1978). *Patterns of attachment: A psychological study of the strange situation.* Hillsdale, NJ: Erlbaum.

Alpert, & Neubauer, P. (1956). Unusual variations in drive endowment. *Psychoanalytic Study of the Child,* 125–163.

American Heritage Dictionary of the English Language. (1992). 3rd. edition, New York: Houghton Mifflin.

American Psychiatric Association. (1987). *Diagnostic and statistical manual of mental disorders* (3rd ed. – rev.). Washington, DC: Author.

American Psychiatric Association. (1988). *Anxiety disorders.* (Division of Public Affairs). Washington, DC: Author.

American Psychiatric Association. (1994). *Diagnostic and statistical manual of mental disorders,* (3rd ed.). Washington, DC: Author.

Ardoin, M. (1990). Bridge of fear. *Tulane Medicine, 21*(3), 17–18.

Babcock, M.L., & Connor, B. (1981, May). Sexism and treatment of the female alcoholic: A review. *National Association of Social Workers,* vol 26(3), 223–238.

Ballenger, J. (1989). Toward an integrated model of panic disorder. *American Journal of Orthopsychiatry, 59,* 284–293.

Barraga, N. (1976). *Visual handicaps and learning.* Belmont, CA: Wadsworth.

Bartenieff, I., & Lewis, D. (1980). *Body movement: Coping with the environment.* New York: Gordon and Breach.

Bartky, C. (1980). *A comparison of the movement profiles of battered, ex–battered, and nonbattered women a pilot study.* Unpublished master's thesis, Hahnemann Medical College, Philadelphia, Pa.

Baum, E.Z., Kluft, R.P., & Reed, L. (1984). Interdisciplinary collaboration in the treatment of MPD: Art therapy, movement therapy and psychiatry (Abstract). In B.G. Braun (Ed.) *Dissociative dissorders: Proceedings of the first international conference on multiple personality/dissociative states.* (91) Chicago: Rush University.

Baum, E.Z. (1991). Movement therapy with multiple personality disorder patients. *Dissociation,* IV:2, 99–104.

Baum, E.Z. (1993). Dance/movement group therapy with multiple personality disorder patients. In E.S. Kluft (Ed. *Expressive and Functional Therapies in the Treatment of Multiple Personality Disorder* (pp. 125–141). Springfield, Il: Chas. C. Thomas.

Beahrs, J. (1982). *Unity and multiplicity.* New York: Brunner/Mazel.

Beck, A.T. (1985). Theoretical perspectives on clinical anxiety. In A.H. Tuma & J. Maser (Eds.), *Anxiety and the anxiety disorders* (pp. 183--196). Hillsdale, NJ: Erlbaum Associates.

Benbow, M. (1977, March). Sensory–motor integration approaches to autism: The tactile system. In J. Brown, (Ed.), *The spectrum of autistic disorders of childhood—Papers presented in honor of the tenth anniversary of the League School of Boston* (pp. 41–47). Boston, MA: Lindemann Mental Health Center.

Benov, R. (1991). *The collected works by and about Blanche Evan.* Available from Blanche Evan Dance Foundation, 146 Fifth Avenue, San Francisco, CA 94118.

Bergman, P., & Escalona, S. (1949). Unusual sensitivities in very young children. *Psychoanalytic Study of the Child,* 3/4, 333–352.

Bettleheim, B. (1967). *The empty fortress.* New York: Free Press .

Black, C. (1981). *It will never happen to me!.* Denver: Mac Publishing.

Blau, B. (1989, March). Pre–play: A modality to foster parent–child interaction with developmentally disabled infants. *Association for Play Therapy Newsletter, 8*(1), 1–3.

Blau, B., & Siegel, E. V. (1978). Breathing together: A preliminary investigation of an involuntary reflex as adaptation. *American Journal of Dance Therapy, 2,* 35–42.

Blume, E. (1991). *Secret survivors:, uncovering incest and its aftereffects in women.* New York: Ballantine Books.

Bowen, N. (1982, December). Guidelines for career counseling with abused women. *Vocation Guidance Quarterly,* 123–127.

Bowlby, J. (1963). *Attachment and loss (Vol. 2): Separation: anxiety and anger.* New York: Basic Books.

Bowlby, J. (1980). *Attachment and loss (Vol. 1): Attachment.* New York: Basic Books.

Bradshaw, J. (1988). *Healing the shame that binds you.* Deerfield Beach, FL: Health Communications.

Bradshaw, J. (1990). *Homecoming: Reclaiming & championing your inner child.* New York: Bantam Books.

Braun, B. G. (1986). *The treatment of multiple personality disorder.* Washington, DC: American Psychiatric Press.

Braun, B.G. (1988a) The BASK model of dissociation, *Dissociation* I:I, 4-23.

Braun, B.G. (1988b) The BASK model of dissociation: Part II - treatment. *Dissociationa* 1:2, 16-23.

Brier, A., Charney, D.S., & Heninger, G.B. (1984). Major depression in patients with agoraphobia and panic disorder. *Archives of General Psychiatry, 41* (11) 29–35.

Brownmiller, S. (1975). *Against our will: men, women and rape.* New York: Bantam Books.

Burlingham, D. (1961). Some notes on the development of the blind. *Psychoanalytic Study of the Child,* 20, 121–145.

Burlingham, D. (1972). *Psychoanalytic studies of the sighted and the blind.* New York: International Universities Press.

Butler, R. (1963). The life review: An interpretation of reminiscence in the aged. *Psychiatry, 26,* 65–75.

Caplow–Lindner, E., Harpaz, L., & Samberg, S. (1979). *Therapeutic dance movement: Expressive activities for older adults.* New York: Human Sciences Press.

Caul, D. (1984). Group and video tape techniques for multiple personality disorder. *Psychiatric Annals,* 14, 50.

Caul, D., Schs, R.G., & Braun, B.G. (1986). Group therapy in treatment of multiple personality disorder. In B.G. Braun (Ed.), *Treatment of Multiple Personality Disorder,* (pp. 143-161). Washington, DC: American Psychiatric Press.

Cermak, T. L. (1985). *A primer on adult children of alcoholics.* Pompano Beach, FL: Health Communications.

Cermak, T. L. (1986). *Diagnosing & treating co–dependency: A guide for professionals who work with chemical dependents, their spouses & children.* Minneapolis: Johnson Institute Books.

Chaiklin, H. (Ed.). (1975). *Marian Chace: Her papers*. Columbia, MD: American Dance Therapy Association.

Chaiklin, S., & Schmais, C. (1979). Chace approach to dance therapy. In P. Bernstein (Ed.), *Eight theoretical approaches in dance–movement therapy*, (pp. 15–30). Davenport, IA: Kendall Hunt.

Chu, J. A. (1988). Ten traps for therapists in the treatment of trauma survivors. *Dissociation, 1*(4), 24–32.

Coons, P.M. & Bradley, K. (1985). Group psychotherapy with multiple personality patients. *The Journal of Nervous & Mental Disease, 173*, 515-521.

Covington, S.S. (1985). *Women and addiction: A collection of papers*. unpublished manuscript La Jolla, CA.

Dell, C. (1970). *A primer for movement description*. New York: Dance Notation Bureau.

Downes, J. (1980). Movement therapy for the special child: Construct for the emerging self. In M. Leventhal (Ed.), *Movement and growth: dance therapy for the special child* (pp.13–17). New York: New York University Press.

Dratman, M. & Kalish, B. (1967, 1971). *Reorganization of psychic structures in autism: A study using body movement therapy*. Paper presented at American Dance Therapy Association Conference, Washington, DC, 1967 and at Bennington College, 1971.

Duggan, D. (1978). Goals and methods in dance therapy with severely multiply handicapped children. *American Journal of Dance Therapy, 7*, 31–34.

Duggan, D. (1981). *Dance therapy*. (Informational brochure available from American Dance Therapy Association, Columbia, MD).

Dulicai, D., & Silberstein, S. (1984). Expressive movement in children and mothers: Focus on individuation. *Arts in Psychotherapy, 11*, 63–68.

Duncan, I. (1927). *My Life*. New York: Horace Liveright

Erfer, T., Goldsand R., & Weinstock, M. (1988, November). Yes! You can do dance/movement therapy with groups of autistic children, within an educational bureaucracy. In *The moving dialogue: A dance between...art, science, politics–Monograph No. 5 and Conference Abstracts of the 23rd Annual Conference of the American Dance Therapy Association* (pp. 102–104). Columbia, MD: American Dance Therapy Association.

Erikson, E. (1968). *Identity, youth and crisis*. New York: Norton.

Evan, B. (1949). *The child's world: Its relation to dance pedagogy*, Article II: "The child's need." [Reprinted in Benov, R. (1991) *The collected works by and about Blanche Evan* (p. 54)].

Evan, B. (1950). *The child's world: Its relation to dance pedagogy*, Article VIII: I am the sun. (Reprinted in Benov, R. (1991). *The collected works by and about Blanche Evan* (p. 80). San Francisco: Blanche Evan Foundation).

Evan, B. (1951). *The child's world: Its relation to dance pedagogy*, Article X The source. ([Reprinted in Benov, R. (1991) *The collected works by and about Blanche Evan* (p. 88)].

Fallot, R.D. (1976). *The life story through reminiscence in later adulthood.* Unpublished doctoral dissertation, Yale University, Department of Psychology, New Haven, CT.

Fisher, S., & Cleveland, S. (1968). *Body image and personality.* New York: Dover.

Fraiberg, S. (1968). Parallel and divergent patterns in blind and sighted infants. *The Psychoanalytic Study of the Child*, 23, 264–300.

Fraiberg, S. (1976). Transcript of discussion. In Z.S. Jastrzembska (Ed.), *The effects of early blindness and other impairments on early development.* New York: American Foundation for the Blind.

Fraiberg, S. (1977). *Insights from the blind.* New York: Basic Books.

Fraiberg, S., & Freedman, D.A. (1965). Studies in ego development of the congenitally blind child. *The Psychoanalytic Study of the Child*, 19, 113–169.

Fraiberg, S., Siegel, B., & Gibson, R. (1966). The role of sound in the search behavior of the blind infant. *Psychoanalytic Study of the Child,* 21, 327–357.

Fraiberg, S., Smith, M., & Adelson, E. (1969). An educational program for blind infants. *Journal of Special Education*, 3, 121–142.

Freud, A. (1965). Normality and pathology in childhood: Assessments of development. In *The writings of Anna Freud* (Vol. 6). New York: International Universities Press. In J. Strackey (Ed. & Trans.).

Freud, S. (1960). *The psychopathology of everyday life.* In J. Strachey (Ed. and Trans.) The standard edition of the complete works of Sigmund Freud (Vol. VI). London: Hogarth (Original work published 1901)

Freud, S. (1964). *New introductory lectures on psychoanalysis*, college edition, J. Strachey (Ed. & Trans.) New York: Norton. (Original work published 1932)

Fuhlrodt, R. (1990). *Psychodrama: Its application to ACOA and substance abuse treatment.* East Rutherford, NJ: Thomas W. Perrin.

Gil, E. (1988). *Treatment of adult survivors of childhood abuse.* Rockville, MD: Launch Press.

Gillman, I. (1980). An object–relations approach to the phenomenon and treatment of battered women. *Psychiatry*, 43, 346–358.

Giovacchini, P.L. (1982). Structural progressions and vicissitudes in the treatment of severely disturbed patients. In P.L. Giovacchini & L.B. Boyer (Eds.), *Technical Factors in the Treatment of the Severely–Disturbed Patient.* New York: Jason Aronson.

Group for the Advancement of Psychiatry. (1968). *Normal adolescence.* New York: Charles Scribner.

Gruber, K.F., & Moore, P.M. (Eds.). (1963). *No place to go: A symposium.* New York: American Foundation for the Blind.

Hammer, E. (1958). *Clinical application of projective drawings.* Springfield: Charles C. Thomas.

Hapeman, L.B. (1967). Developmental concepts of blind children between the ages of three and six as they relate to orientation and mobility. *International Journal for the Education of the Blind, 17,* 41–48.

Hartman, C., & Burgess, A. (1988). Information processing: A case application of a model. *Journal of Interpersonal Violence, 3* (2), 28-34.

Herman, G., & Renzurri, J. (1978). *Creative movement for older people.* Hartford, CT: Institute for Movement Exploration.

Herman, J. (1981). *Father–daughter incest.* Cambridge, MA: Harvard University Press.

Hinsie, L.E., & Campbell, R.J. (1974). *Psychiatric dictionary* (Fourth Edition). New York: Oxford University Press.

Horowitz, M.S., Wilner, N., Kaltreider, N., & Alvarez, W. (1980). Signs and sysmptoms of post-traumantic stress disorder. *Archives of General Psychiatry, 37,* 85-92.

Huston, K. (1984). Ethical decisions in treating battered women. *Professional Psychology: Research and Practice, 15*(6), 822–832.

Ibrahim, F. A., & Herr, E. L. (1987, January). Battered women: A developmental life–career counseling perspective. *Journal of Counseling and Development, 65,* 244–248.

Jarvis, R. (1991, July/August). Panic attacks: Recognition and management. *Journal of the American Academy of Physician Assistants, 4* (5), 373-382.

Johnson, T. (1988). Children who act out sexually. In J. McNamara, J. W. Kerr, & R. Judy (Eds.), *Fostering the sexually abused child.* Knoxville, TN: University of Tennessee College of Social Work.

Kalish, B. (1968). Body movement therapy for autistic children—A description and discussion of basic concepts. *Proceedings of the 3rd Annual Conference of the American Dance Therapy Association* (pp. 49–57). Columbia, MD: AMerican Dance Therapy Association

Kanner, L. (1955). *Child psychiatry.* Springfield IL: Charles C Thomas.

Kasl, D.C. (1989). *Women, sex and addiction.* New York: Harper & Row.

Kaufman, E. (1989). The psychotherapy of dually diagnosed patients. *Journal of Substance Abuse Treatment, 6,* 9–18.

Kernberg, O.F. (1975). *Borderline conditions and pathological narcissism.* New York: Jason Aronson.

Kestenberg, J. (1985a). The role of movement patterns in diagnosis and prevention. In D. A. Shaskan & W. L. Roller (Eds.), *Paul Schilder: Mind explorer.* (pp. 97–160). New York: Human Sciences Press.

Kestenberg, J. (1985b). The flow of empathy and trust between mother and child. In E. J. Anthony & G. H. Pollack (Eds.), *Parental influences: In health and disease.* (pp. 137–163). Boston: Little Brown.

Kestenberg, J. (1975). *Children and parents.* New York: Jason Aronson.

Khantzian, E. J. (1985). The self–medication hypothesis of addictive disorders: Focus on heroin and cocaine dependence. *American Journal of Psychiatry, 142*(11), 1259–1264.

Khantzian, E. J. (1986). A contemporary psychodynamic approach to drug abuse treatment. *American Journal of Drug and Alcohol Abuse, 12*(3), 213–222.

Khantzian, E. J., Halliday, K. S., & McAuliffe, W. E. (1990). *Addiction and the Vulnerable Self.* New York: Guilford Press.

Kluft, E.S. (1993). A literary overview of multiple personality disorder. In E.S. Kluft (Ed.), *Expressive and Functional Therapies in the Treatment of Multiple Personality Disorder* (pp. 3-22.) Springfield, IL: Charles C. Thomas.

Kluft, R.P. (1983). *Childhood antecedents of multiple personality.* Washington, DC: American Psychiatric Press.

Kluft, R.P. (1984a). An introduction to multiple personality disorder. *Psychiatric Annals,* 4, 19-24.

Kluft, R.P. (1984b). Treatment of multiple personality disorder: A study of 33 cases. *Psychiatric Clinics of North America,* 7, 9-29.

Kluft, R.P. (1987). An update on multiple personality disorder: A study of 33 cases. *Psychiatric Clinics of North America,* 7, 9-29.

Kluft, R.P. (1991). Multiple personality disorder. In A. Tasman & S.M. Goldfinger (Eds.), *American Psychiatric Press Review of Psychiatry* (pp. 161–188). Washington, DC: American Psychiatric Press.

Knight, R. P., & Friedman, C.R. (Eds.). (1954). *Psychoanalytic psychiatry and psychology.* (pp. 97–109). New York: International Universities Press.

Kohut, H. (1971). *The analysis of the self.* (pp. 153–163). New York: International Universities Press.

Kohut, H. (1977). *The restoration of the self.* New York: International Universities Press.

Kramer, S. (1991). Psychopathological effects of incest. In S. Kramer & S. Akhtar (Eds.), *The Trauma of Transgression: Psychotherapy of Incest Victims* (pp. 3-12). Northvale, NJ: Jason Aronson.

Krystal, H. (1977). Aspects of affect theory. *Bulletin of the Menninger Clinic, 41,* 1–26.

Krystal, H. (1982). Alexithymia and the effectiveness of psychoanalytic treatment. *Journal of Psychoanalytic Psychotherapy, 9,* 353–388.

Laban, R. (1960). *The mastery of movement* (2nd ed.). London: MacDonald and Evans.

Laban, R., & Lawrence, F. C. (1947). *Effort*. London: MacDonald & Evans.

Lamb, W. (1965). *Posture and gesture*. London: Gerald Duckworth.

Landy, R. (1986). *Drama Therapy* . Springfield, II: Charles C. Thomas

Landy, R. (1993). *Persona and Performance*. New York: Guilford.

LaPlanche, J., & Pontalis, J.B. (1973). *The language of psychoanalysis*. New York: Norton.

Leventhal, F., & Chang, M. (1991). Dance/movement therapy with battered women: A paradigm of action. *American Journal of Dance Therapy, 13*(2),131–145.

Leventhal, M. (1981). *An overview of dance therapy for the special child*. Workshop presented at Laban/Bartenieff Institute of Movement Studies, New York City

Levin, J.D. (1991). *The treatment of alcoholism and other addictions*. Dunmore, PA: Jason Aronson.

Levy, F.J. (1979). Psychodramatic movement therapy: A sorting out process. *American Journal of Dance Therapy, 3*(1), 32–42.

Levy, F.J. (1988). *Dance movement therapy: A healing art*. Reston, VA: American Alliance for Health, Physical Education, Recreation and Dance.

Levy, F.J. (1992). *Dance movement therapy: A healing art*. Reston, VA: American Alliance for Health, Physical Education, Recreation, and Dance.

Levy, S. (1950). Figure drawing as projective test. In L.E. Abt & L.Bellak (Eds.), *Projective psychology*. New York: Knopf.

Levy, S. (1958). Symbolism in animal drawings. In E. Hammer (Ed.), *Clinical application of projective drawings*. Springfield, IL: Charles C. Thomas.

Lewis, E. (1983). The group treatment of battered women. *Women and Therapy, 2*(1), 51–58.

Lewis, P. (Ed.). (1984). *Theoretical approaches in dance–movement therapy*, Vol. II. (2nd ed.). Dubuque, IA: W.C. Brown–Kendal/Hunt Publishing.

Lewis, P. (Ed.). (1986). *Theoretical approaches in dance–movement therapy*, Vol. I. Dubuque, IA: W. C. Brown–Kendal/Hunt Publishing.

Lewis, P. (1993). *Creative transformation: The healing power of the arts*. Wilmette, IL: Chiron Publications.

Lewis, P., & Loman, S. (Eds.). (1990). *The Kestenberg movement profile: Its past, present applications and future directions*. Keene, NH: Antioch New England Graduate School.

Lewis, P., & Loman, S. (1992). Movement components of affect: Tension–flow attributes within the Kestenberg Movement Profile (KMP). *American Dance Therapy Association 27th Annual Conference Proceedings*. Columbia, MD: American Dance Therapy Association.

Loman, S. (1991). Refining movement interventions in dance/movement therapy: A model of nonverbal interaction utilizing the Kestenberg Movement Profile (KMP)

system of movement analysis. In *Shadow & light: Moving toward wholeness.* Columbia, MD: American Dance Therapy Association.

Loman, S., & Brandt, R. (Eds.). (1992). *The body mind connection in human movement analysis.* Keene, NH: Antioch New England Graduate School.

Machover, K. (1949). *Personality projection in the drawing of the human figure.* Springfield, IL: Charles C. Thomas.

Mackay, B. (1989). Drama therapy with female victims of assault. *Arts in Psychotherapy, 16,* 293–300.

Mahler, M. (1970). *On human symbiosis and the vicissitudes of individuation.* New York: International Universities Press.

Mahler, M. S., Pine, F., & Bergman, A. (1975). *The psychological birth of the human infant: Symbiosis & individuation.* New York: Basic Books.

Marlatt, G.A., Baer, J.S., Donovan, D.M., & Kivlahan, D.R. (1988). Addictive behaviors: Etiology and treatment. *Annual Review of Psychology, 39,* 223–252.

Masterson, J. (1972). *Treatment of the borderline adolescent: A developmental approach.* New York: Wiley Interscience.

McDougall, J. (1991). *Theaters of the mind: Illusion and truth on the psychoanalytic stage.* New York: Brunner/Mazel. (Original work published in French, 1982).

McMahon, A.W., & Rhudick, P.J. (1967). Reminiscing in the aged: An adaptational response. In S. Levin & R. Kahana (Eds.). *Psychodynamic studies on aging* (pp. 64–78). New York: International Universities Press.

McNamara, J. (1989). *Tangled feelings.* Ossining, NY: Family Resources.

McNamara, J., & McNamara, B. H. (1990). *Adoption and the sexually abused child.* Portland, ME: Human Services Development Institute.

Meekums, B. (1991). Dance movement therapy with mothers and young children at risk of abuse. *Arts in Psychotherapy, 18,* 223–230.

Merman, H. (1990). The use of precursors of effort in dance/movement therapy. In P. Lewis & S. Loman (Eds.). *The Kestenberg movement profile: Its past, present applications and future directions.* Keene, NH: Antioch New England Graduate School.

Mills, R.J. (1970). Orientation and mobility for teachers. *Education of the Visually Handicapped, 2,* 80–82.

Missildine, W.H. (1963). *Your inner child of the past.* New York: Simon & Schuster.

Mittelman, B. (1954). Mobility in infants, children and adults. *Psychoanalytic Study of the Child 9,* 284–319.

Mittelman, B. (1957). Mobility in the therapy of children and adults. *Psychoanalytic Study of the Child 12,* 284–319.

Mnukhin, S., & Isaev, D. (1975). On the organic nature of some forms of schizoid or autistic psychopathy. *Journal of Autism and Childhood Schizophrenia, 5* (2), 99–108.

Moore, B., & Fine, B. (Eds.). (1968). *A glossary of psychoanalytic terms and concepts.* New York: American Psychoanalytic Association.

Moreno, J.L., & Moreno, Z.T. (1975). *Psychodrama: Action therapy and principles of practice* (Vol. III). New York: Beacon House.

Moreno, Z.T. (1966). Psychodramatic rules, techniques and adjunctive methods. *Psychodrama and Group Psychotherapy Monographs* (p. 41). New York, Beacon House.

Morrison, M. (1986). A conspiracy of silence. *Journal of the Medical Association of Georgia, 15*(8), 480–481.

Murphy, J. (1979, October). The use of non–verbal and body movement techniques in working with families with infants. *Journal of Marital and Family Therapy, 5*(4), 61–66.

Needler, W., & Baer, M. (1982). Movement, music and remotivation with the regressed elderly. *Journal of Gerontological Nursing, 8,* 497–503.

Nemiah, K. (1980). Dissociative disorders. In H. Kaplan, A. Freedman, & B. Sadock. (Eds), *Comprehensive Textbook of Psychiatry,* 3rd ed., (pp. 1544-1561). Baltimore, MD: Williams & Wilkins.

New York City Public Schools—Division of Special Education. (1991). *Educational services for students with handicapping conditions.* New York: New York City Board of Education .

NiCarthy, G. (1982). *Getting free: A handbook for women in abusive relationships.* Seattle: Seal Press.

North, M. (1972). *Personality assessment through movement.* Boston: Plays, Inc.

Padus, E. (1986). Uncertainty: Public stressor number one. In *Your emotions and your health,* (pp 193—196). Emmaus, PA: Rodale Press.

Paley, A. N. (1988). Growing up in chaos: The dissociative response. *American Journal of Psychoanalysis, 48,* 72–83.

Peluso, E., & Peluso, L. (1988). *Women and drugs: Getting hooked, getting clean.* Minneapolis, MI: CompCare Publishers.

Pope, J. (1991, April 10). Panic: An interview with Earl Campbell. *Times Picayune,* pp. 1, 8.

Putnam, F.W. (1989). *Diagnosis and treatment of multiple personality disorder.* New York: Guilford.

Putnam, F.W., Guroff, J.J., Siberman, F.K., Barban, I. & Post, R.M. (1986). The clinical phenomenology of multiple personality disorder: Review of 100 recent cases. *Journal of Clinical Psychiatry, 47,* 285-293.

Reicher, D. (1990). *Primary prevention and early intervention.* Unpublished manuscript.

Rifkin–Gainer, I. (1991). An interview with Blanche Evan. *American Journal of Dance Therapy, 5.* (Reprinted in Benov, R. (1991). *The Collected Works by and about Blanche Evan* (p. 192). San Francisco: Blanche Evan Foundation).

Rifkin–Gainer, I., Bernstein, B., & Melson, B. (1984). *Dance movement work therapy: The methods of Blanche Evan.* in P. Bernstein, (Ed.), *Theoretical approaches in dance–movement therapy*, (Vol. II). Dubuque, IA: Kendall/Hunt.

Romer, G., & Sossin, K. M. (1990). Parent–infant holding patterns and their impact on infant perceptual and interactional experience. *Pre– and Post–Natal Psychology Journal, 5*(1).

Rounsaville, B., Lifton, N., & Bieber, M. (1979). The natural history of a psychotherapy group for battered women. *Psychiatry, 42,* 63–78.

Ruttenberg, B., Kalish, B., Wenar, C., & Wolf, E. (1977). *Behavior rating instrument for autistic and other atypical children.* Chicago : Stoelting.

Ryan, J. (1989). Victim to victimizer: Rethinking victim treatment. *The Journal of Interpersonal Violence, 4*(3), 325-341.

Ryan, J. (1990). Sexual behavior in childhood. In J. McNamara & B. H. McNamara (Eds.), *Adoption and the sexually abused child.* Portland, ME: Human Services Development Institute.

Samuels, A. (1973). Dance therapy for geriatric patients. *Proceedings of the Eighth Annual Conference of the American Dance Therapy Association,* 8, pp.27–30.

Sandel, S. (1978). Reminiscence in movement therapy with the aged. *Arts in Psychotherapy, 5*(4), 217–22.

Sandel, S., Chaiklin, S., & Lohn, A. (Eds.). (1993). *Foundations of dance/movement therapy : The life and work of Marian Chace.* Columbia, MD: The American Dance Therapy Association.

Sandel, S., & Johnson, D. (1987). *Waiting at the gate: Creativity and hope in the nursing home.* New York: Harworth Press.

Schechter, S. (1987). *Guidelines for mental health practitioners in domestic violence cases.* Washington, DC: National Coalition Against Domestic Violence.

Schilder, P. (1950). *The image and appearance of the human body.* New York: International Universities Press.

Schmais, C. (1974). Dance therapy in perspective. In K. Mason (Ed.), *Dance therapy focus on dance VII* (pp. 7–12). Reston, VA: American Alliance for Health, Physical Education, Recreation and Dance.

Schmais, C. (1985). Healing processes in group dance therapy. *American Journal of Dance Therapy, 6,* 17–36.

Schmeck, H. (1988, June 7). New research cites brain abnormalities as factors in autism. *The New York Times* , p. c3.

Schreiber, F.R. (1984). *Sybil.* New York: Warner.

Sechehaye, M.A. (1951). *Symbolic realization.* New York: International Universities Press.

Smith, A. W. (1988). *Grandchildren of alcoholics: Another generation of co–dependency.* Deerfield Beach, FL: Health Communications.

Spiegel, D. (1984). Multiple personality disorder as a post-traumatic stress disorder. *Psychiatric Clinics of North America,* 7: 101-110.

Spitz, R. (1965). *The first year of life.* New York: International Universities Press.

Stern, D. (1977). *The first relationship: Mother and infant.* Cambridge: Harvard University Press.

Stern, D. (1985). *The interpersonal world of the infant: A view from psychoanalysis and developmental psychology.* New York: Basic Books.

Stern, D. (1990). *Diary of a baby.* New York: Basic Books.

Subby, R. (1987). *Lost in the shuffle: The co–dependent reality.* Deerfield Beach, FL: Health Communications.

Summit, R. (1983). The child sexual abuse accommodation syndrome. *Child Abuse and Neglect, 7,* 177–193.

Terr, L. (1990). *Too scared to cry.* New York: Basic Books.

Terry, W. (1956). *The dance in America.* New York: Harper & Brothers.

Toda, S., & Fogel, A. (1993). Infant's response to the still face situation. *Developmental Psychology, 29*(3), 532–538.

Victor, G. (1983). *The riddle of autism—A psychological analysis.* Lexington, MA: Lexington Books.

Walker, L. (1979). *The battered woman.* New York: Harper and Row.

Walker, L. E. A. (1989). Psychology and violence against women. *American Psychologist, 44,* 695–702.

Wallace, B. C. (1989). Relapse prevention in psychoeducational groups for crack cocaine smokers. *Journal of Substance Abuse Treatment, 6,* 229–239.

Waterman, J., Kelly, R., McCord, J., & Olivieri, M. (1990). *Reported ritualistic and nonritualistic sexual abuse in preschools: Effects and mediators.* Department of Psychology, University of California–Los Angeles Research and Educational Institute, Harbor UCLA Medical Center: Los Angeles, CA.

Wegscheider–Cruse, S., & Cruse, J. (1990). *Understanding co–dependency.* Deerfield Beach, FL: Health Communications.

Whitfield, C. L. (1987). *Healing the child within: Discovery & recovery for adult children of dysfunctional families.* Deerfield Beach, FL: Health Communications.

Wing, L. (Ed.). (1976). *Early childhood autism—Clinical, educational, and social aspects* (2nd ed.). New York: Pergamon Press.

Winnicott, D.W. (1965). *The maturational process and the facilitating environment.* New York: International Universities Press.

Winnicott, D. (1971). *Playing and reality.* New York: Basic Books.

Wurmser, L. (1974). Psychoanalytic considerations on the etiology of compulsive drug abuse. *Journal of the American Psychoanalytical Association, 22,* 820–843.

Wurmser, L. (1978). *The hidden dimension: Psychodynamics in compulsive drug use.* New York: Jason Aronson.

Contributors

Fran J. Levy, Ed.D., B.C.D., C.S.W., (Board Certified Diplomate Clinical Social Work), ADTR, Editor, is the author of *Dance/Movement Therapy: A Healing Art* (AAHPERD, 1988). Dr. Levy has a private practice in Brooklyn, NY where she directs The Center for the Arts in Psychotherapy. Dr. Levy is a Fellow in the American Society for Group Psychotherapy and Psychodrama and in the Clinical Society for Social Work Psychotherapists. Her doctorate is in Creative Arts Therapy from Rutgers University. Levy has been teaching the integration of the arts in psychotherapy for the last 25 years.

Judith Pines Fried, M.A., ADTR, Co-editor, former faculty member at Immaculate Heart College and Loyola Marymount University in Los Angeles; she shared a studio with Jane Manning for 10 years in California, where she conducted a private practice. Fried now lives in New York City where she is recognized for her skills as an editor, writer, and poet.

Fern Leventhal, M.A., ADTR, Co-editor, has been involved since 1976 in the field of dance therapy as a clinician, teacher, supervisor, and author. She has taught at both Pratt Institute and the College of New Rochelle. Ms. Leventhal is presently a doctoral candidate in Counseling Psychology at Teachers College, Columbia University, and is employed by the New York University Medical Center.

Edith Z. Baum, M.A., ADTR, is a dance/movement therapist with over 15 years of clinical experience. She works at the Institute of Pennsylvania in Philadelphia. Since the opening of the Dissociative Disorder Unit in 1989, she has been working exclusively with Multiple Personality Disorder patients.

Bonnie Bernstein, M.Ed., ADTR, M.F.C.C., was mentored by Blanche Evan, 1970–1982. She is a therapist, teacher, supervisor, and consultant and is affiliated with several Rape Crisis Centers. She researched therapeutic dance in West Africa and Malaysia and has a private practice in Palo Alto, California.

Bette Blau, M.A., ADTR, has been a movement therapist since 1971. She has lectured and taught in graduate movement therapy and special education programs and has published in a variety of journals and books. Currently, she is Director of Movement Therapy Services at Little Village School in Long Island, NY, where she supervises therapists and interns.

Meg Chang, M.S., ADTR, is Assistant Professor and Coordinator of the Graduate Dance/Movement Therapy Specialization at Lesley College in Cambridge, MA. She has facilitated community and shelter support groups for battered women and their children, and is also a staff consultant in shelters for domestic violence. Ms Chang also operates a private practice.

Diane Duggan, M.A., ADTR, doctoral candidate, New York University, has been professionally involved in the field of dance therapy as a clinician, supervisor, teacher, and author since 1973. She has taught at Hunter College and New York University Her work has been presented at the annual American Dance Therapy Conference.

Tina Erfer, M.S., ADTR, works within the New York City Public School system and is in private practice. She supervises and trains dance therapists and frequently presents her work at professional conferences. She is past President of the NYS Chapter of the American Dance Therapy Association.

Steve Harvey, Ph.D., ADTR, RDT, RPT, is a licensed psychologist working privately with young children and their families in Colorado Springs, CO. He is registered by the national dance, drama, and play associations. He teaches and consults on family issues involving abuse and adoption throughout the United States and Europe.

Amy Scott Hollander, M.A., received a master's degree in movement, from Wesleyan University. Ms. Hollander is the Director of the Alzheimer's Day Program, St. Camillus Health Center, Stamford, CT, and President, Fairfield County Alzheimer's Association.

Susan Kierr, M.A., ADTR, studied psychology at Wellesley and Columbia University, taught dance at The Boston Conservatory, and wrote *The Overeaters, Eating Styles and Personalities.* She received her Master's in Expressive Therapy from Lesley College and she has worked in rehabilitation medicine, education, and psychiatry.

Joan Lavender, Psy.D., M.A., is a Psychoanalytic Psychotherapist with a certificate from the Institute for Contemporary Psychotherapy. She has her doctorate in Clinical Psychology from Widener University and has recently completed a postdoctoral fellowship in psychotherapy research from the State University of New York in Brooklyn. She is in private practice.

Eileen M. Lawlor, C.I.S.W., C.A.D.C., ADTR, is a Clinical Social Worker and Creative Arts Psychotherapist in private practice. Specializing in addiction/co-dependency and trauma work, she serves as adjunct faculty at the University of Connecticut's West Hartford campus in the School of Social Work.

Susan Loman, M.A., ADTR, is currently the Director of the Dance/Movement Therapy Program at Antioch New England Graduate School. The co-editor of two volumes related to the Kestenberg Movement Profile (KMP), she has been teaching the KMP system of movement analysis for 10 years.

M. Barbara Murray-Lane, M.A., M.S.W., ADTR, has worked extensively for the past 13 years in the psychiatric and substance-abuse field with women and children. She maintains a private practice, specializing in dissociative disorders, substance abuse, and women's issues.

Debra Reicher, Ph.D., received her doctorate from the California School of Professional Psychology, Los Angeles, in 1990. She has extensive experience working with infants, young children, and their caregivers. She is Director of the adolescent psychiatric program at Van Nuys Hospital in southern California and is also in private practice.

Sherry Rose, M.A., ADTR, is a psychotherapist and educator in New York City, where she also continues to privately supervise dance/movement therapists. She has been working in the field of chemical dependency since 1987, as a clinician, trainer, curriculum developer, and substance-abuse counselor educator. She received analytic training at the New York Center for Psychoanalytic Training, and teaches addiction and human service courses as an Adjunct Assistant Professor at the City University of New York. Currently, she is attending the Master's program in Public Health at Hunter College.

Susan L. Sandel, Ph.D., ADTR, is the Clinical Coordinator of Long-Term Mental Health Services at Veterans' Memorial Medical Center, Meriden, CT. She is a faculty member at the University of New Haven and co-author of *Waiting At the Gate: Creativity and Hope in the Nursing Home.*

Wendy Sobelman, M.P.S., ADTR, received her Master's from Pratt Institute in 1981. She is a Senior Clinician, Dance Therapist at St. Luke's-Roosevelt Hospital in the personality disorders unit of the Day Treatment Center in New York City. She supervises staff and students and is in private practice.

Index

158, 163, 196-199, 226, 233
Body image, definition, 49, 151
Borderline personality
  See also case examples/vignettes
  characteristics, 69-71, 78-79, 81, 82
  definition, 69
  genesis, 71
  treatment, 78, 80-81
Boundaries, 32-33, 110
Bowen, N., 63
Bowlby, J., 77, 121, 169, 181
Bradley, K. 86
Bradshaw, J., 94, 109, 111
Brandt, R., 213
Braun, B.G., 9, 84-86
Break dance, 235-236
Brier, A., 126
Brownmiller, S., 50
Buie, D.H. 69
Burgess, A., 122
Burlingham, D., 151-152
Butler, R., 139

Campbell, R.J., 151
Caplow-Lindner, E., 137
Case examples/vignettes
  adopted children/Sandra, 170-180
  aged, 139-143
  anxiety disorder, 124-130
  attachment disorder, 183-189
  autism, 202-207
    Warren, 216-223
  battered women, 45-57
  blind children/Sue & Jon, 153-163
  borderline personality, 70-82
  See also Multiple Personality
  Disorder/Multiplicity
  co-dependency/Jessie, 111-117
  co-dependency, 109-114
  learning impaired adolescents/Tommy &
  Trudy, 236-240
  multiple personality disorder, 88-90
  See also Multiplicity
  multiplicity, Nameless/Rachel, 10-40
  See also Multiple Personality
  Disorder
  sexual abuse, 45-57

Sandra, 167-180
substance abuse, 94-99, 104-107
Catharsis, 54, 61
Caul, D., 86
Cermak, T.L., 110
Chace, M., 138, 197-198, 208, 231
Chaceian circle, 226
Chaiklin, S., 135, 197-198, 231
Chang, M., 62
Charney, D.S., 126
Chemical addiction, *See also* substance
  abuse
Chemical dependency, 126
Child abuse, 8
  effect, 89
  See also case examples/vignettes, sexu-
  al abuse/adopted child
Child development, 8
Chu, J.A., 66
Cleveland, S., 49
Co-consciousness, 9
Co-dependency
  See also case examples/vignettes
  definition, 109
  in infancy, 110
  patient characteristics, 110
  therapy, 109
Confrontation, 112-113
Connectedness, 9, 21
Connor, B., 94
Consciousness, 9
Constancy, 19, 24, 28
Containment, of movement, 104
Conversion symptoms, 242
Coons, P.M., 86
Costumes, use of, 233, 237-238
Countertransference, 66-67, 81
Courchesne, 194-195
Covington, S.S., 94
Creative art therapy, 7, 10, 168
Creative arts therapists, 10
Creative dance, 44, 51, 56, 65
Creative expression, 19
Creative improvisation, 76
Creative intervention, 8
Creative movement, 61, 133
Creative transformation, 79